A DIFFERENT KIND OF CARE

A Different Kind
of Care

The Social Pediatrics Approach

GILLES JULIEN, MD

Translated by Kathe Lieber

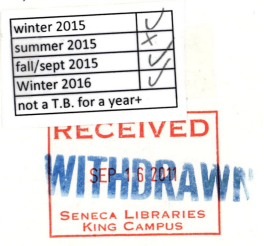

Published for the Montreal Children's Hospital
by
McGill-Queen's University Press
Montreal & Kingston · London · Ithaca

© McGill-Queen's University Press 2004
ISBN 0-7735-2800-8 (cloth)
ISBN 0-7735-2801-6 (paper)

Legal deposit third quarter 2004
Bibliothèque nationale du Québec

Printed in Canada on acid-free paper that is 100% ancient forest free
(100% post-consumer recycled), processed chlorine free.

McGill-Queen's University Press acknowledges the support of the
Canada Council for the Arts for our publishing program. We also
acknowledge the financial support of the Government of Canada
through the Book Publishing Industry Development Program (BPIDP)
for our publishing activities.

National Library of Canada Cataloguing in Publication

Julien, Gilles, 1946–
    A different kind of care: the social pediatrics approach/Gilles Julien;
translated by Kathe Lieber.

    Translation of: Soigner différemment les enfants.
    Includes bibliographical references.
    ISBN 0-7735-2800-8 (bnd)
    ISBN 0-7735-2801-6 (pbk)

    1. Pediatrics – Social aspects. 2. Children – Health and hygiene –
Social aspects. 3. Children with social disabilities – Health and hygiene –
Case studies. 4. Children – Diseases – Prevention – Social aspects.
I. Lieber, Kathe II. Montreal Children's Hospital. III. Title.

RJ47.7.J8513 2004   618.92   C2004-901847-7

This book was typeset by Dynagram Inc. in 10/13 Baskerville.

Contents

Acknowledgments

I would like to thank some important colleagues whose inspiration, encouragement, and technical support have enabled me to write this book. Very special thanks go to Claudette Everitt, a community health nurse whose support and constant presence have been an integral part of the Assistance aux Enfants en difficulté (AED) project in the Hochelaga-Maisonneuve neighbourhood of Montreal. Claudette has certainly seen the great suffering of our young patients but can also testify to the renewed sense of hope the project has brought to many families.

Thanks go as well to the following colleagues, a constant source of motivation and support in our work, who give us the strength to go on: Dr Gloria Géliu, a pediatrician and professor at Ste-Justine Hospital, who has been a hands-on inspiration in everything I have done and a totally reliable source of information; Jacques Lorion, director general of the CLSC Côte des Neiges, a man with a great big heart, whose confidence gives us wings; Dr Vania Jimenez, a great friend and support in all my work with children; Dr Christine Collin, Suzanne Descôteaux, and Lucie Côté, who kindly read the manuscript and gave me their extremely useful comments.

I would also like to thank the following colleagues for reading this manuscript (or perhaps I should say decoding and transcribing it): Colette Laredo of the CLSC Côte des Neiges, and Sylvie Belisle and Claudette Lemay, both of the Outaouais regional health board. The Outaouais public health department also provided support for the publication of this book. All profits from the sale of this book go to the AED project.

I am extremely grateful to the administrators of the Department of Pediatrics at the Montreal Children's Hospital and to the MCH Foundation for believing in this book and deciding to make it available as a training tool for professionals who work with children. Special thanks go to Dr Harvey Guyda for his ongoing commitment to the project and to Dr Anne Marie MacLellan for her efficient and sustained interventions.

Finally, I would like to express my deepest gratitude to Dr Nick Steinmetz, who wrote the foreword to this book. For many years, he has provided tremendous moral support and motivation for my work in social pediatrics.

Gilles Julien, MD

Foreword

We value the care, protection, and development of children, and with good reason. Vulnerable for many years, they need our protection. Attaining maturity and competence in our increasingly complex world is a lengthy process that requires education and prolonged guidance.

As individuals, we take care of our children because we love them, and because we see our life flow into theirs. They carry our genetic heritage into the future. We intuitively feel what the Tao teaches: "In thy offspring, thou art born again. That, mortal, is thy immortality."

As a society, we value children because they ensure continuity. Beyond mere survival, society has an interest in children being healthy, capable, competent, and responsible. We continue to engineer our physical and social environment to protect children from abuse, prevent injury and illness, heal them when they are sick or injured, and offer education to all. While we take pride in these successes, the consequences of a new phenomenon have, until quite recently, escaped our attention: the progressive and dramatic urbanization of our society.

With urbanization has come a different form of poverty, unlike the poverty seen in the village or rural setting. Urban poverty brings dependence, isolation, disruption of family and breakdown of social cohesion. In turn, this results in loneliness and the loss of a sense of self-worth, control, and parenting skills. The absence of support and guidance, along with comforting, understanding, positive role models, too often brings violence, abuse, abandonment, and failure at school. The wisdom of the African proverb "It takes a whole village to raise a child" no longer operates.

The health and welfare of children has been an important concern of physicians for a long time. About one hundred years ago, physicians began to identify the care of children as being worthy of particular and increasingly exclusive attention. Advances in technology and in our understanding of physiology, biochemistry, genetics, nutrition, and physical and psychological development have brought us progressively to the practice of twenty-first-century pediatrics – in offices, clinics, and hospitals. That expertise now goes beyond physicians to include nurses, social workers, child-life workers, teachers, police officers, and judges.

Social and medical measures have had a tremendous impact. In our society, a child's death is rare and serious illness is uncommon. However, the increasing number of children suffering the effects of poverty now exceeds the number of children affected by cancer or kidney disease – or any other recognized malady treated in our major pediatric medical centres. And these children do not usually show up at the doctor's office or the hospital. They show up in police stations, in court, in youth protection centres – and they are absent from school.

Dr Gilles Julien is one of a growing group of alert, passionate, and committed physicians who have taken note of the rising number of children manifesting the corrosive effects of poverty. He has shown how these children fall between the cracks of the many bureaucratic jurisdictions that are funded to assist them. Taking a low-tech, inexpensive, and humane approach, he has shown how the quiet and persistent application of existing knowledge through often simple gestures can have decidedly spectacular results.

In this book, Dr Julien describes a framework within which we can understand and address these issues. He challenges us to focus on the child's needs and set aside traditional roles and limiting regulations, attitudes, and practices.

A true pioneer in our midst, Dr Julien has shown himself to be courageous and persistent, as well as endlessly creative. But be warned – this unrestricted, selfless, and natural expression of love in daily life is not for the faint of heart.

Nicholas Steinmetz, MD, MPH, FRCP(C)
Associate Professor of Pediatrics,
Epidemiology, and Biostatistics
McGill University

Introduction

Here we are in the third millennium, yet so much still remains to be done for our children. Although we have (in theory) improved child protection by making declarations and passing legislation at the provincial, national, and international levels, child poverty is rising and children's rights often seem to be an illusion, even in relatively wealthy countries like Canada. At every level of society, children seem to be increasingly isolated. And with isolation come insecurity and neglect – all serious impediments to the development of children.

In my pediatric practice over the past quarter-century and more, children have always been central to my concerns. Every day, I see children from all types of backgrounds. Some are spoiled in economic terms, while others lack the bare necessities of life. Each child is different, special, and endearing in his or her own way. Some are gentle, others shy or fearful, some distant or confrontational, some are sick in body or in mind. These are the children who often suffer in silence – or cry out to be heard, but no one is listening. All children have a little light burning bright in their eyes and their hearts. That spark means that there is something we can do to ease their suffering before it is too late.

For many years, my pediatric practice has centred on children who suffer from conditions that appear quite complex to practitioners. These are the children who do not get the care they need in busy clinics, the "problem" children who are frequently labelled and abandoned by the system. It was for them that I wrote this book – to give them a voice, so they will be heard at last. These children are my inspiration and my motivation.

The social pediatrics approach enables us to relieve children's suffering and cure illnesses that may seem complex in terms of modern medicine. In some cases, all that modern medicine has to offer is the short-term relief of prescription drugs. This book begs to differ, presenting an approach that wanders a little from the beaten path. The objective of social pediatrics is to promote a compassionate relationship, composed in equal parts of listening and empathy, involving the therapist, the child, the family, and the community. This approach is straightforward, effective, and accessible to all. It provides some pathways and solutions for everyone who has an interest in giving children what they need to grow and develop in health and happiness.

This book is divided into two parts. Part One discusses the foundations of social pediatrics. What is in the child's best interest from a global health perspective? What roles do society, health-care professionals, teachers, and families have to play? How do living conditions and other factors affect children's development? What are the major problems children experience today, especially the problems that we find most difficult to solve? What basic elements do children need for good health?

Part Two tells the stories of some troubled children, defining the practice of social pediatrics in real life. I do not pretend to have all the answers to children's problems. I simply want to share my experience and make a humble contribution to the well-being of our children. Their stories are deeply touching. Why does Dennis keep on losing weight? Why does Max never cry, though anyone can see how sad he feels? What about Robert, who's been trundled from one foster family to the next? Why is Christine still not talking at the age of seven? Why is Ahmed so passive?

I believe that we can find ways to give these children real relief from their suffering. And we must, because the future of our society depends on the well-being of our children.

A DIFFERENT KIND OF CARE

After a month or two a pediatrician was called in. "The child is exhausted," he said, and gave me a dose of cod liver oil. Nobody ever asked me why I couldn't sleep, nor why I always carried Argus's gnawed ball around with me.

Susanna Tamaro, *Follow Your Heart*

PART ONE

The Theory of Social Pediatrics

Before you were conceived, I wanted you
Before you were born, I loved you
Before you were here an hour, I would die for you
This is the miracle of life.

Maureen Hawkins, *The Miracle*

Health is not brought with a chemist's pill nor saved by the surgeon's knife. Health is not only the absence of ills, but the fight for the fullness of life.

Piet Hein, *Prologue at the Celebration of WHO's 40th
Anniversary in Copenhagen*

Social pediatrics is a term used to describe the importance of caring for children in a way that reflects the social context in which they live. The term encompasses everything that relates to the child, society, and the community. It provides a much-needed link to *preventive and curative health care and social services* by taking a global approach that considers the child as a whole person in a specific context.

Taking concrete steps to support the development, health, and well-being of children is a logical progression from scientific knowledge, based on special sensitivity to children and an acute sense of the need for balance in their living environment. From all this comes the concept of a more social, more community-based approach that centres on the child, his or her overall needs, living conditions, and environment. So we must rethink our traditional models of

practice to serve children and their families in ways designed
to meet their needs more effectively in terms of their health
and well-being. These services are integrated, not comp-
artmentalized. Health programming is not imposed from
"outside" but created and put together with the children
themselves and those in their milieu according to their
needs, abilities, and expectations, and set against a backdrop of respect and autonomy.

Social pediatrics is based on a simple method of meeting
children's needs. It closely resembles the instincts that guide
all attentive parents in terms of meeting their children's
everyday needs for food, sleep, or play. It is much the same
technique that parents use to decide whether their baby's
cries mean happiness, sadness, fear, or pain. The main thing
is to listen and to sense what children are saying, beyond
their external appearance and symptoms. Once that is done,
the program of services comes easily.

For example, a child may be angry because he has a strong
temperament or because he is sincerely offended, but more often than not, anger conceals a much deeper suffering that cannot be expressed in any other way. An analogy can be made
with a feverish child who has an ear infection or pneumonia –
we need to find out what the problem is before we can bring
down the fever and avoid a further decline in health.

This method is accessible to everyone, within the limits of
their responsibility for the child. It can be used by parents,
who are duty-bound to provide for their child, or by doctors
and nurses, social workers and other professionals working
with the child, who have a duty to provide treatment. It can
be used by teachers, who have a duty to provide an education, and by adults in the community, whose role is to provide support and guidance.

OBSERVE, LISTEN, AND UNDERSTAND

To prevent problems and support children, or deal with situations that put their health and well-being in jeopardy, we
need to learn to free up all our senses, to *observe and listen*.

In *L'influence qui guérit*, ethnopsychiatrist Tobie Nathan states that a symptom can be considered a text without a context.[1] Therapeutic activity invariably involves discovering the context in which the text of the symptom can be made coherent (understandable and absolutely necessary). Nathan stresses the importance of finding out what is really happening, beyond external manifestations. We must try to *understand* by going beyond the children's symptoms (remember the example of the anger and the fever and what was behind them), finding out which emotions are involved and taking a real interest in children, their friends and family, and how they see things.

This method involves letting the children take the lead, immersing yourself in the dynamics of the human beings so that you can detect their strengths and weaknesses, decode different messages that may be buried deep, and help the children activate healing mechanisms that will restore peace and balance.

Listening, understanding, and taking *effective action*: most professionals certainly possess the competence and sensitivity to listen and understand. All too often, however, the resulting action is piecemeal, fleeting, and imperfectly adapted. This is what we call "band-aid solutions" – solutions that provide immediate relief but only on a temporary basis.

Supporting children and their families to ensure a lasting state of health through sustained action with the assistance of the community – this is what's at stake in social pediatrics. But people from different segments of society need to commit to acting together. Politicians need to come up with a social contract that includes a range of political, economic, and fiscal changes. Managers need to refocus the objectives of their institutions to provide services adapted to children and families. Health-care professionals need to commit to shared action with resources in the community. Every bit counts, and it all adds up when it comes to achieving our final objective: healthy children.

WHAT IT TAKES

There are three basic steps to follow in applying this approach in real life:

1 Collect all the essential information, starting with "secrets": the child's own stories, motivations, confidences,
  and family secrets.
2 To obtain this privileged information, you need to enter
  the child's world – at home and at school. Bear in mind
  that information of an intimate nature must be elicited in
  a climate of confidence and privacy, which is much easier
  to do in the child's own familiar surroundings.
3 The general attitude of the interviewer, regardless of position, title, or habits, must reflect a high level of open-
  mindedness and great respect for the child and those in
  the child's circle.

Six Steps to Follow

A truly effective social pediatrics intervention is a six-step
process.

1 First and foremost, display an attitude of openness and let
  the child take the lead for this introductory session.
2 Be on the lookout for every possible tangent, indicator, sign,
  and symbol you can pick up from the child and family.
3 Listen attentively to what the child tells you. These
  confidences are usually short and surprising.
4 Move around, shift places, play with the child – in other
  words, establish your relationship by getting closer to the
  child.
5 Discuss ideas and hypotheses with those involved, testing
  out your own theories and asking for further information
  as needed. Explore various ways of explaining conditions
  and coming up with lasting solutions.
6 Focus on what the interview accomplished. Decide who
  does what and what role each person should play, set dead-
  lines, and decide what steps will be taken to follow up and
  what role the network has to play.

The main thing is to connect with the core of the child –
what remains when you've finished peeling away the things

that don't really matter. Once you've analyzed the outer lay-
ers of the child – temperament, development, habits, beliefs, and behaviours – you can go straight to the deeper
aspects – the child's roots, core, and belonging.

The central idea is "Tell me where you come from and I'll
tell you who you are." Once you succeed in touching the
very heart of the person, you have access to a being who
is wide open, receptive, and motivated for the balancing
process.

Basically, this method involves an updated version of the
traditional scientific method – collecting and analyzing data,
setting forth several hypotheses, and formulating a plan that
will be followed and evaluated along the way. For the sake of
clarity, let's call it the EEDA method.

E is for ESTABLISHING a special relationship. This involves
   getting to know each other, entering each other's world,
   starting to feel comfortable, and establishing a cooperative
   footing that is conducive to assistance and support. This step
   and the next both involve collecting data. The first step is
   best conducted at home, at school, and in the child's surroundings, with his or her family or caregivers, so that sharing can take place.

E is for EXCHANGING. Each person is open to the others, without any preconceived ideas on the facts, ideas, and emotions
   attached to the child. Exchanging views on beliefs and habits
   and dealing with different ways of doing things are indispensable to better understanding.

D is for DECODING. This means analyzing knowledge and experience in an integrated way to decode the meaning of the
   problem or disease and decide what action to take next.

A is for ACTION. Steps to take to enhance the child's well-being
   are spelled out, and causes and needs are identified in a true
   consensus between professionals and family members. The
   best way to achieve successful, effective intervention is to take
   action based on needs that are understood, accepted, and
   considered a priority by all the parties, using a range of
   adapted tools.

The EEDA approach applies to all children and can be used by everyone who works with children. For example, it would work with an eight-year-old who is displaying aggressive behaviour towards his parents, teacher, or little sister, helping the child define the feelings of anger that are disturbing him and shedding light on his behaviour and his emotions, way down deep.

This approach can help us understand what emotional injury is at the root of such a strong impulse at this particular stage in the child's development. In this case, it helps us come up with steps that will set in motion long-lasting problem-solving mechanisms. The approach is also intended for the one-year-old who has stopped gaining weight and having regular bowel movements and seems determined to die. With the EEDA approach, we can try to find an explanation for the deep sadness that haunts this baby, causing him to toss and turn even though he hasn't learned to walk or talk yet. It will also help us with the boy who, at the age of five, finds no enjoyment in life and wonders why he was born.

A great deal remains to be done to help children suffering from social disorders and those who have been victimized by society. The EEDA method really works for all those children who have been hurt, betrayed, or abandoned, who are crying out from despair and suffering, as reflected in functional problems, diseases, or developmental disorders.

CHAPTER ONE

The Best Interests of the Child

A SHARED RESPONSIBILITY

The importance society places on children has varied greatly over the centuries, even from decade to decade, and certainly from culture to culture. As societies change and evolve, social contexts shift and we see similar shifts in the degree of interest various societies take in their children. The role, value, and importance of children are dynamic concepts, rising or falling along with socioeconomic or political indicators. In the best interests of the child, we must give families every chance to fill their role fully, rather than leaping in to replace them at the first opportunity. Only parents can give their children the continuity that an ever-changing society is unable to guarantee.

On the international scene, the children of war are a heart-rending example. According to UNICEF, children caught in the crossfire account for a high proportion of the more than two million children who have been murdered, four to five million who have been maimed, 12 million who have been left homeless, the million or more who have been orphaned, and the ten million suffering from psychological traumas – from 1985 to 1995 alone.[1] Many wars and conflicts fought on the backs of children and without paying them any heed spring to mind. In recent years, they include

Rwanda,[2] Yugoslavia, Iran, Iraq, Algeria, and many other countries where horrors have been committed against children. Not to mention famines, landmines, forced separations, and migrations, which cause all kinds of trauma for children, who far from being spared are frequently the victims of societies in distress.

Public opinion, which carries a certain collective moral weight, remains sensitive to the suffering endured by the children of the world, (sometimes) loudly proclaiming its revulsion and indignation. Happily, our collective conscience retains a certain ethical standard that, at least in theory, guarantees the best interests of the child. More specifically, we can see this on the local scene when a sensational event, such as a case of sexual violence, neglect, infanticide, or pedophilia, triggers reactions of blazing indignation in the newspapers and in the public forum.

Despite the fluctuating forms that the victimization of children takes in our society and around the world, we must acknowledge that society still cherishes the principle of defending the best interests of the child. Historically, through all the chaos and the trauma, it is mainly communities and families that have supported and protected children in a relatively consistent manner[3]. We can nearly always count on the commitment and responsibility of adults, parents, and friends to act as advocates and staunch defenders of the best interests of the child, come what may.

CREATING FAVOURABLE CONDITIONS

When it comes to local resources, we need to create child-friendly conditions if we hope to avoid the kind of irreparable trauma that jeopardizes the development and lives of children. We must seek from the parents (a term we will define below) the love and strength required to foster the best interests of the child. Parents in turn must be able to rely on the extended family to support them as they care for their children. And we must look to the community for adapted resources so that we can offer the range of tools and services it takes to raise a child to adulthood.

Not long ago, I was visiting a family that was trying to cope with a five-year-old who had grown progressively more obnoxious and violent since the age of two. The parents were in despair and on the verge of throwing up their hands, broken-hearted. The child had already been suspended from school and daycare, and babysitters refused to look after him. The child himself was in extreme distress, the father was depressed, and the mother, in constant tears, was thinking of leaving.

The first foundations of a solution were to be found in the immediate family. The grandmother, who was present for the home visit, and the aunt had already decided to call a family council to stop the situation from deteriorating further and to support the parents, who were at their wits' end. The local respite centre and recreation department would set things in motion to help the child and divert him from this dangerous trajectory. Later on, more specialized resources would be called in if necessary. In this case, it took a bit of a push to set off the natural mechanism that was lagging behind. The main thing that was needed was a good dose of support and confidence in the strengths of the family, which had not yet dared to mobilize to help the child.

Speaking of the best interests of the child, we must stress the role of significant adults – adults who are important to the child, who are there at the right time to help, guide, and care for the child, or even temporarily to replace the parents in hard times. They are primarily found in the family (blood usually is thicker than water) but sometimes also in the family circle, among the neighbours or community resources. Significant figures are helpful to both children and parents in that they can provide help and relief in complete confidence, without any preconceptions, out of the goodness of their hearts. They are the most valuable partners of children and parents alike, those who can provide the most consistency next to the parents themselves.

Professionals who work with children and families must learn to recognize the issues involved in the child's best interests, as well as the limitations of the concept at a time when societies are in a state of flux and legislation governing the general well-being of children is subject to a wide range of interpretations.[4]

The commitment proclaimed by a society that wants the best for its children is certainly modulated by various contingencies and major upheavals; as a result, it fails to offer the necessary consistency. On the other hand, we generally find such consistency of commitment and interest among those who are responsible for children – in particular the parents, despite their own problems. The best person to work for the well-being of children is the parent or other responsible adult who has a personal and emotional involvement with the children, who will prove to be an indefatigable ally, sometimes needing support, but whose motivation is unquestionable.

At this point it is crucial to stress that to our mind, the concept of parent and family means those individuals who have the most direct and closest connection with the child, those who serve as guide, helpmate, role model, and protector. The term *parent* generally refers to the natural parent, playing his or her role to the fullest extent. But it may also mean a substitute parent, generally a significant adult, relation by marriage, foster parent, or someone else who, whether temporarily or on a full-time basis, takes on the job in the absence or incapacity of the natural parent. Similarly, the broader concept of the *family* includes not only the immediate family (father and mother, brothers and sisters) but also relations by marriage and, frequently, neighbours and community resources.

The Parent-Child Relationship and the Role of Society

The winning equation in the best interest of children lies in the parent-child or adult-child relationship that lasts for their whole lives. This is doubtless the most reliable and stable, selfless, and most productive relationship in terms of supporting the child's well-being. In general, parents will flee from war to protect their children, deprive themselves to put food in their children's mouths, and face the worst to give their children a brighter future.

Acting in the best interests of the child therefore means having confidence in the parents, who can, more than anyone else, ensure the well-being of their children. Society or the government must play a role in establishing conditions that are "family-friendly," so that families can play their roles fully and support them in times of trouble. Children are generally nestled under the protective wing of their parents, who in turn are supported by the community and their family circle and encouraged by society. This is in the best interest of the child because the child's needs are better expressed and respected by a functional family that can freely and consciously respond without interference. In this context, the state's contribution is to preserve the integrity and functionality of the family.[5]

Functional authority is first of all the authority of the parents or an adult (more often than not a family member) who is most likely to show sufficient sensitivity to the child. This involves offering protection, compassion, and education, finding basic mechanisms for the child's harmonious development, and providing access to the tools needed to build the child's physical, sociocultural, and spiritual integrity.

The complex phenomenon of child development requires an ongoing relationship between children and parents. This sort of constant interaction establishes an *attachment*, that state of reference that is so essential to learning, understanding, and developing, and later to *autonomy*, the capacity to control your impulses and affects and become a sociable being. In order to develop, the child must also be motivated; that motivation comes to a large extent from the dynamic interaction between parent and child.

To achieve this complex interaction, the family needs to feel free to act in a climate in which it can experience true intimacy. Anything that gets in the way of family intimacy, experience, ways of doing things, or beliefs will disrupt the intimacy of the parent-child relationship and therefore deter the development of the child. Any betrayal of family intimacy or the need for autonomy in terms of the child's development can disrupt the formation or maintenance of attachments, again jeopardizing the development of the child.

The Role of the State

If we acknowledge the importance of parental ability in ensuring the development and protection of children in the fragile developmental stages, then we must also recognize the limitations of certain parents. It does happen that parents have innate or acquired limitations that hinder their capacity to support the child fully until he or she achieves autonomy. Sometimes "hard knocks" can derail the parents from their fundamental supportive role. In some situations, the responsible adult may lose his or her sense of values, leading to neglect, violence, exploitation, or abandonment. One way of protecting the child involves removing the child temporarily from the family if the family is placing the child's security or development at risk. In extreme circumstances, the government may intrude on family intimacy in the best interests of the child.

However, such fundamental – even sacred – values as the primacy of the parent's role cannot be touched except with great delicacy and infinite precaution. So great an intrusion into family life can only be justified in unacceptable situations in which the well-being, integrity, and safety of the child are placed at risk. Under such circumstances, the state may attempt to provide a better environment for the child – one that is more secure and can compensate for what is lacking in the family.

The state can try to do better, but success in this endeavour, as we all know, is quite rare. It may prove difficult to find significant adults or caregivers for the child, there may be a lack of continuity in the network, or the child may encounter neglect or even violence in government-operated facilities. Sometimes the state only aggravates the situation, making things even more difficult for the child and family once they are separated. That is why the intrusive intervention of the state should not proceed from personal or professional judgments that promote one way of doing things, or one socio-cultural vision, over another. The only situation in which it is justifiable to invade the privacy of the family and undermine the child's right to independent parenting is when the child's human rights are being infringed – that is, when the child's well-being and safety have actually been compromised. The entire procedure, moreover, must take place in an ethical manner, with respect for and confidence in the restoration of the parents' independent role and the privacy of the family.

In 1989, after lengthy efforts, the United Nations released a statement called *The Convention on the Rights of the Child.* This ground-breaking gesture reaffirmed on the world stage the principle of the "best interests of the child," stating clearly that the principle must transcend the care given to children[6] and support those who have responsibility – the family. The principle of the best interests of the child must take priority in all interventions, whether it be the prescription of medication, hospitalization, or when the child's integrity is at risk as in cases of child abuse or neglect. Adherence to this principle alone ensures the child's overall well-being in a context of full equality and justice. The same principle underlies interventions in social pediatrics that look out for the best interests of the child, acting in close partnership with the parents and the family circle.

CHAPTER TWO

The Child in Context

WHAT CHILDREN NEED

What children really need has not changed over the centuries. What has changed dramatically is the social context. Technology marches on, but children remain extremely vulnerable. However, risk factors, especially factors of a psychosocial nature, have increased exponentially, and it is not at all rare to find several such factors in the same child. This makes the child even more vulnerable and even more likely to develop "modern" health problems, such as adjustment disorders that lead to serious problems like delinquency, drug abuse, and suicide.

The needs of children, as stated by Gustavson during the preparation process for the *United Nations Convention on the Rights of the Child*, fall into six categories[1]:

1 the need to have roots – an identity or base;
2 the need to be considered a full-fledged human being;
3 the need to receive attention from adults in general;
4 the need to have parents;
5 the need to have relationships with significant adults;
6 the need to have a future.

All these needs address a single goal: to give children *an identity of their own*, so that they feel a sense of belonging to

parents, a community, and a culture throughout their lifetime, but most importantly during the early years of life, the
most active developmental period. Identity basically refers
to the context of the child – the child's meaning, motivation, and future.

It is essential for everyone to be able to identify with a family, a place, and a way of life that reflects and colours an individual's persona. In many cultures, the importance of identity
is demonstrated by rites and customs that the community
considers to be of paramount importance. There are special
rites to welcome and name the child, and to mark milestones:
birth, first steps, and times of transition. These rites are all
part of the process of identifying the child.

In North America, for example, First Nations peoples traditionally welcome a child with various ceremonies attended by
the entire community, a symbolic gesture of great significance. The Inuit have a longstanding tradition of marking
the child's place in the community by investing the child with
the identity of an ancestor, who will protect and accompany
the child throughout his or her life. In Africa, some tribes believe that a child is a complete being, but starts out as a
stranger. To ensure the child's well-being and survival, special
identification procedures are carried out to welcome, acknowledge, and name him or her.

Ethnopsychiatrist Tobie Nathan has given some thought to
the concept of identity and filiation – the importance of ver-
tical and horizontal links for every human being. Nathan's
work on this and many other topics is most enlightening.
Here is an excerpt: "Moses was doubtless the greatest of the
Jewish poets. His position of primacy could have led him to
imagine that he was the only father of his son, the only father
of all his descendants. God came down to teach him that a
child with only one filiation, a child without affiliation, is a
dead child, son of a dead father."[2]

Identify is fragile by its very nature. Children from all types
of backgrounds who experience major trauma, whether
through neglect or abandonment, or by being marginalized
at an early age, are at high risk of losing the mechanisms that

regulate filiation or affiliation. When parents are absent, for example, or where there are no parents, or when they are preoccupied with survival or the production of material possessions, they cannot reproduce the systems that are needed for the balanced development of their children. They spoil them, "buying" them with material possessions, isolating them in their rooms with their own TVs or Nintendo games, or they give the children to someone else to raise or ignore them completely. No child can develop properly under such conditions; survival is the best one can hope for. So it is necessary to take preventive action to redress the balance in these children, reflecting the precious system of identity that defines the person. Adults are responsible for seeing that the child's needs are met. While this is first and foremost a parental and familial responsibility, it is also a social, moral, and political responsibility.

THE CHILD'S CIRCLE: FAMILIES, ADULTS, SOCIETIES

The family as an influential unit has undergone immense changes in recent decades. Families have been greatly affected by the high divorce rate, socioeconomic changes, and the redefinition of women's and men's roles within the home and beyond its walls. The role of parents has also changed greatly in terms of their presence, consistency, availability, and the very nature of the parent-child bond. The likelihood that a family will be affected by divorce has risen from seven percent in 1960 to over fifty percent today, which means that one in two children will be forced to live with a single parent, generally the mother, for at least some time[3].

During the past 30 years, the number of couples living together before marriage and the number of common-law marriages have also risen substantially. Although fathers tend to be more involved in their children's lives than in previous generations, their involvement frequently becomes more marginal after separation and divorce. The amount of money available is often significantly reduced once the parents divide their assets,[4] and this has a direct impact on the children's quality of life.

It is generally agreed that one in four Canadian children is living in poverty. A 1997 Statistics Canada survey reported that a solid majority (seventy-one percent) of children raised by single mothers were living in families whose incomes were at or below the low-income cut-off line. A more recent survey confirms this trend.[5] Poverty is certainly a negative determinant for health, largely because of the multiple stress factors it adds to the family's load. But it is also clear that families in a better financial situation are not exempt from problems that affect children. Children's problems cannot be attributed to poverty and single-parent families alone.

Changes in the family as an institution have meant that children must adjust to new situations. Whether they lose special contact with one or both parents, experience identity problems thanks to separation, break-up, or other family trouble, or suffer the byproducts of poverty, children are the losers, and the net effect is an increased level of vulnerability and exposure to a wide range of risks.

LIVING CONDITIONS AND CHILD DEVELOPMENT

Illness is not linked to chance, but to something in our social, economic and cultural environment ... In an individual's social, economic and cultural environment are found some of the most recognized secrets for longevity and good health. In particular, the techniques a person uses to cope with the stresses of life are fundamental. These techniques are associated with self-esteem and a feeling of control, two factors that vary in direct correlation with socio-economic status[6].

A study dating back to 1956 showed the importance of the social context in child development by analyzing the rise in repeat hospitalizations due to poor housing conditions[7].

Difficult environments can certainly have a negative impact on child development, but it is clear that the way children respond to this type of risk depends on and is modulated by their gender, age, stage of development, and overall living conditions[8]. There appears to be a dynamic relation between temperament, baggage, experience, and environment that determines the extent to which a child is vulnerable or resistant to risk factors. While one child living under difficult conditions will suffer from developmental delays, another, living under identical conditions, will develop in a harmonious manner.

According to a 1994 Statistics Canada report, the risk factors that have the greatest impact on the development of children are lack of social support for the family, family dysfunction, and depression of the parents. The combined effect of several factors appears to be even more harmful in developmental terms.

It is also important to consider the repercussions of living with parents who have difficulty coping with their child's developmental stages. In the first two years of a child's life, the impact of this is felt mainly in social or cognitive development – the ability to form links with other people and perform many learning tasks. In the period from two to five, the impact falls mainly on the child's behaviour[9]. In other words, the effects of risk factors on the child are somewhat modulated according to the child's stage of development. It is extremely important to bear this in mind when we try to understand reactions in children that are otherwise difficult to decode, inform parents of the risks their children are exposed to under certain circumstances, and take preventive action.

Amazingly, for a certain group of children, exposure to negative environments does not seem to produce any noticeable problems, whether physical, emotional, or behavioural. To all appearances, they are free of the negative effects generally observed in other children living under similar conditions. Observing the resistance some children have to adversity has led to the concept of *protective factors*, which to some extent counterbalance the risk factors to which these children are exposed. That resistance is what we call "resilience."

Those who work with children need to recognize what makes them vulnerable and what serves as a protective factor. Vulnerability factors increase the risk of and potential for the appearance of various problems or symptoms. Inversely, the protective mechanism reduces the risk of and potential for developing problems. This partly explains children's wide range of reactions and the variable impact negative circumstances can have on their development.

THE RISK FACTOR

The concept of the risk factor[10] is well known, along with the litany of conditions and incidents that have a negative impact on children's health: poverty, being raised in a single-parent family, family problems, a difficult temperament, abuse, and neglect being the most commonly recognized factors. Risk factors may be personal, originating in the family, or related to the environment. What really counts, however, is the nature and intensity of the risk in relation to the individual over time. In and of itself, a risk has no particular significance. For example, being poor does not necessarily place a person at risk. It all depends on the circumstances and intensity of the risk, how long it lasts, and the cumulative effect of various risks. This group of elements makes children more vulnerable, with potentially catastrophic effects on their development. It all depends as well on their personal abilities, *previous experience*, developmental stage, and level of tolerance. There also appears to be a tolerance threshold,[11] lower for some and higher for others, up to which the child can resist disagreeable events. Even in wartime or in situations of great terror, children who are direct victims show different levels of tolerance in their adjustment and in the consequences they suffer.

Other Influential Factors

Various other attributes will influence children's vulnerability or protect them when they have to cope with negative environments. *Previous experience* is one aspect that influences vulnerability in the sense that children, like all humans, are already "sensitized" by previous negative experiences. It is as if a child who has previously been exposed to such problems as maltreatment, loss or cruelty, for example, becomes more sensitive to other negative events, which in turn set off more intense negative reactions in the form of developmental or behavioural problems. A parallel can be drawn with a hypersensitive reaction (e.g., an allergy) whereby a subject is sensitized to a food, for example, and then has a violent reaction to the same food the next time. Similarly, a child who has previously been exposed to severe distress or been a witness to violence will have a strong reaction under certain circumstances, displaying extreme, uncontrollable sorrow or excessive, deep anger. These difficult events from the past appear to be "buried" in the child and become "latent risks," ready to resurface when the child is exposed to new risks.[12]

For example, we know that sexual violence in childhood can be harmful to social interactions in adulthood or raise the risk of depression when other types of social problems arise. The same is true for loss and grieving, which have a cumulative effect over the years, becoming a risk factor for emotional problems later on. Based on these examples, we could say that the concept of accumulated risk serves as a counterbalance to the concept of thresholds of tolerance, varying from child to child. This is another fundamental notion that should be kept in mind by everyone who hopes to work effectively with children.

Gender and *temperament* also have an impact on how vulnerable a child will be. Boys seem to be more sensitive than girls to family conflicts and more likely to develop secondary problems related to emotions and behaviour. Girls, on the other hand, seem to be more sensitive than boys to multiple

losses over the long term, which tends to result in consequences of a psychological nature.

Temperament can help us to understand the mechanisms
that provoke behavioural reactions to environmental influences. Temperament can be defined as the sum of the child's
daily behaviours as expressed in three modes: the *emotion
mode,* or the ability to cope with an event even under stress;
the *sociability mode,* the ability to form relationships with others and cooperate; and the *action mode,* which refers to the
sum of physical activities.[13] Every child possesses all three
modes, and the modes make up the child's temperament. For
example, a seven-year-old with a difficult temperament who
shows a high level of emotivity, poor socialization, and hyperactivity, may be at high risk of developing behavioural problems around the age of 12.

The state of vulnerability and protective factors are crucial
to understanding children's needs. The resilience typical of
some children – their ability to deal with sad or difficult
events without sustaining emotional wounds – is not yet well
understood. In an excellent article, Garnezy[14] suggests a series of psychosocial variables that can help parents and professionals understand or predict children's resistance in the
face of adversity. The variables are as follows:

- personality traits, such as independence, self-esteem, and
  positive social orientation;
- a warm, consistent family, with parents who are not having
  problems;
- the availability of support outside the family, encouraging
  and reinforcing the child's efforts.

These variables form the foundation of the ability to resist,
and probably also play a role in raising the threshold of tolerance to stress-producing events in the environment. That
ability is certainly dynamic and subject to many other factors
during its development that determine the mechanisms and
processes that help the child negotiate the hazards and

pitfalls that lie ahead. It becomes a prerequisite for building and preserving the child's health.

These theoretical considerations are borne out in a clinical setting. We frequently observe children who, despite many difficulties in their environment and despite adversity, manage to survive and develop "normally." These children nearly always have a light shining from within, as reflected in shining eyes, a magnetic personality, a curiosity about the world, and a desire to learn and communicate. That topic will be discussed in greater detail in Part Two of this book.

SITUATIONS THAT PLACE CHILDREN AT RISK

Poverty. While social pediatrics focuses on children in general, its specific focus is children living in situations or contexts that place them at risk. Conditions associated with poverty are important factors in the children's environment, affecting their future and the way they develop. There is also a recognized link between poverty (and the poor living conditions that go with it) and child morbidity and mortality.

Household income is a fundamental indicator of a child's well-being, and many studies have shown that children who grow up in low-income families tend to get lower grades in school and are less successful in the labour market.

The Encarta Dictionary definition of poverty is "the state of being poor ... not having enough money to take care of basic needs such as food, clothing, and housing." The very real poverty that affects children is harmful because it attacks a whole set of factors that determine their well-being: their diet is not sufficiently nutritious; they live in unhygienic conditions; they don't get enough exercise or recreation. This is the lot of many children who do not have access to healthy living conditions, and there is a direct correlation with material or financial poverty. A more insidious hidden form of poverty resulting from social or cultural inequities targets the most vulnerable in society, frequently women and children.

It is the result not only of insufficient means but also of ghettoization and lack of access to the basic tools and services that allow for harmonious human development. This kind of poverty involves a whole set of social, material, and cultural inequities of which certain individuals or groups tend to be the victims, which have a negative impact on their development and their future. In Canada, to repeat, approximately one in four children live below the official poverty line.

What is the real scope of the more general poverty that affects Canadian children, and more importantly, what are the trends that lead to such impoverishment? These are the necessary questions we must ask to understand the new morbidities that affect children and adolescents. Poverty declined somewhat in the 1950s and 1960s in many countries, but the poverty rate has rebounded since the 1970s, specifically among certain social groups.[15] In Canada, generally speaking, poverty seems to have stabilized somewhat, but in recent years disparities have continued to grow. So much for all the politicians' grand promises to eradicate poverty by the year 2000 through social programs.

Regardless of trends or countries, however, the immutable fact remains that children are the population group most affected by poverty – and the most likely to be victimized by poverty. Cuts in social services, which we now see on an ongoing basis, affect children more: fewer services plus reduced access to services equals a decline in well-being. Is this in the best interests of children, as decreed by the *Convention on the Rights of the Child?*

Lack of access to health care. In a study on access to health-care services, researchers found that poor children had fifty percent less *access* than other children to a source of regular care or even acute care.[16] In other words, it was more difficult for poor children to obtain any form of care than it was for their more fortunate counterparts. In addition, it has been shown that poor children do not benefit from *continuity* of care, in terms of either going to the same site for care or consistently seeing the same health-care providers. This phenomenon of disparate and dysfunctional care is well known in impoverished areas and is recognized as a negative determinant (i.e., risk factor) for the health of children, leading to physical ailments (e.g., asthma or repeated earache) as well as psychosocial problems (manifest in a tendency to throw tantrums, for example, or run away, or in other behavioural problems, etc.). These are the very problems, of course, that require continuity and coherence in terms of treatment and follow-up. Without access and continuity, there is no point in "thinking prevention" for poor children and others. The entire support system for children is at stake when these conditions are not met. In one of the world's most sophisticated and expensive health-care systems, a large number of children do not have access to basic preventive care. Those who do have access do not necessarily receive the same quality of care as their better-off counterparts. This is why social pediatrics targets the most vulnerable groups of children – it is simply a matter of justice and equity.

Clearly, health is not a priority for many children and families living in conditions of extreme poverty,[17] since their main goal is simply to survive. First of all, they need to put food on the table every day and find and keep adequate housing and a steady source of income. The extremely precarious state of these families, their isolation from social activities and the community, and their permanent state of exclusion compromise any relationships they might have with a health-care system that is itself fragmented and not sufficiently adapted in many cases. A child with an acute health problem will receive prompt but partial service. When it comes to overall health care, adapted service will not be truly available, since access is frequently impossible and continuity is unthinkable under such conditions. Efforts have been made in some communities to give poor families somewhat better service through partnerships developed between local interveners and families and community groups and non-governmental organizations to develop adequate services. Such initiatives are, however, rare and fragile, since it is usually very difficult to obtain funding. A prime example in Quebec are the local community service centres, known by their French initials, CLSCs. CLSCs were developed to meet the local needs of children but over time they have lost this specific mandate due to increasing health costs and increased emphasis on the needs of outpatients and the elderly. Services now appear to be uneven and are frequently left in the hands of professionals alone.

Poor children are sicker than their better-off peers and more often affected by various health problems. High rates of infant mortality, premature babies and low birthweights, accidents, delayed growth, iron deficiency (anemia), lead poisoning, and hearing loss are frequently their fate.[18] These conditions, most of which are preventable, cause children's health to decline, compromising their development today and for the future and reducing their chances of escaping poverty. The physical, emotional, and intellectual consequences of these problems are enormous and often become permanent if they are not checked.[19]

Low-birthweight babies (under 2,500 grams) are a striking example. This condition and its consequences are the factors most frequently associated with perinatal and infant mortality, and there is a direct correlation with socioeconomic status.[20] Respiratory problems, delayed growth, and accidents also occur more frequently among poor children. This may be an indirect correlation, however, and more closely linked to conditions of poverty, such as reduced access to good food, greater exposure to pollution (industrial or domestic) like cigarette smoke, living in more unsafe surroundings, or having parents who are less "available." The net effect remains indisputable – poor children are more liable to have headaches, bronchitis, upper respiratory obstructive disorders, and accidents than other children.[21]

The World Health Organization recognizes two ways of explaining the effects of poverty on children's health.[22] The organizational explanation is related to low income and lack of access to resources. The other, more dynamic explanation involves parents' health habits and their impact on the health of their children. Whichever explanation we choose, we must avoid making value judgments and blaming the victims for their poor state of health, which leads to a failure to take the necessary steps to improve the overall health of children, who must live with a status that is not of their own choosing.

Harmful environments. Studies have shown that lifestyle habits, rather than socioeconomic status, are responsible for the precarious health of poor children. In a study on pregnancy, Brooke et al.[23] reported that mothers who smoke were the main factor in low birthweights and that socioeconomic factors did not appear to play a significant role in this case. Other studies[24] have concurred that the *smoking mother* is a major determinant of differing mortality rates between social classes, even going so far as to suggest that political programs designed to improve living conditions for the poor may not be effective in reducing inequities in health status.

We must avoid taking a limiting, distrustful view of the poor that could lead to coercive attitudes or policies in which the victim becomes responsible for her own misfortunes, rather than a more global perspective of promoting health in a way that is designed to support the parents, not render them powerless and hold them responsible for their condition.

Lifestyle habits and behaviours associated with health are evidently directly related to the social environment and to socioeconomic possibilities and constraints that modulate risk factors and protective factors when it comes to children's health. Promoting healthy living habits (among them quitting smoking, especially by pregnant women) is certainly a good way to help reduce inequities, but if such a solution stands in the way of taking steps to improve living conditions and reduce poverty, it will be a barrier to preventive approaches that can help reduce the effects of poverty on health status.

To take effective action against these negative impacts on the health and development of children, we need to act globally at the social, political, and community levels. Although health-care services have a relatively marginal effect, they can make a notable difference as long as they remain accessible, acceptable, and adequate. We will discuss below what this means and how such services must involve the parents if they are to be effective – handing power back to the parents and respecting their integrity and abilities. "We must do everything we can to improve the skills and behaviours of those who are disadvantaged ... There is consensus on several success factors, including continuity, intensity, stability, flexibility, and early introduction of services and programs, which are as essential as a global approach, community participation, teamwork, and ongoing cooperation between professionals and the administration."[25]

Mistreatment of children. The *mistreatment* of children causes illness and suffering, impeding their development and wellbeing. A child who is chronically mistreated will sustain injuries in every sphere – physical, emotional, and intellectual. The child may react through hyperactive or aggressive behaviour, withdraw into a morose state, or suffer from uncontrollable headaches or persistent sleep problems. The child's whole life will be disrupted, with enormous, lifelong repercussions on his or her development. A child who feels devalued or belittled as a result of mistreatment or unhealthy family conflicts will lose self-confidence and feel powerless. The child will be tempted to run away, to lash out at others to provoke rejection – in fact, to provoke.

The mistreatment of children[26] takes various forms, all of which lead to severe social and emotional handicaps. *Neglect* is the most common and most insidious form of mistreatment. Neglect means failing to give the child the attention every child absolutely must have, whether that means physical attention (poor food, failing to protect the child from danger) or emotional attention (indifference and rejection).

Physical abuse involves the use of abusive force on the child, based on a model of abuse of power. *Emotional abuse* moves from deprecation and intimidation to exploitation and rejection, all of which diminish the child's nature. *Sexual abuse* involves the flagrant exploitation of the child's naivety and immaturity, frequently by making threats and using force. "In his destitution, the child gives an adult who is not self-assured a sense of power, and is moreover very often his sex object of predilection."[27]

The mistreatment of children is invariably an exercise of power by the adult over the child, with flagrant failure to respect the child as a person. It does not only occur in the home; it may also happen at school, in the street, and with friends and caregivers. Any adult can potentially mistreat a child.

The effects of mistreatment are extremely severe, depriving children of the sense of safety and love they need as they grow up. Every incident of mistreatment reveals an attitude of spitefulness, deprecation, and hatred towards the child.[28] No wonder we see such distress in every child who has been mistreated in some way.

Children who have been the victims of mistreatment frequently feel sad and have little interest in playing with their peers. Their confidence and self-esteem are low, and some experience growth problems that can be irreversible. Others present with complications related to brain damage, either neurological problems or developmental disorders (e.g., language delays) or learning problems (e.g., lack of progress at school). On the emotional level, behavioural problems are frequently observed, such as hyperactivity or aggressive behaviour. A good number of delinquents or adult rapists or abusers were themselves mistreated as children. Intellectual delays also frequently appear to be the consequence of mistreatment. The impact of sexual abuse in particular depends on the origin, duration, and intensity of the abuse, with consequences that can prove to be catastrophic in terms of the child's long-term development and psychological integrity.

The origin of mistreatment. According to the scientific literature, socioeconomic and sociocultural changes are directly
related to the incidence of mistreatment of children. Upheavals relating to major changes in society particularly affect cultural values and habits and have a direct impact on
family integrity. These changes cause enormous stress, frequently associated with the impoverishment of surroundings
and individuals. It should come as no surprise that family environments are becoming more and more fragile. As family
situations become more precarious, the effects are felt in
terms of the care children receive: with adults less available
to them, they become increasingly victimized. This description reflects the current evolution of our society and the
growing number of children who are victims of mistreatment
at every level of society. And it explains why a more socially
oriented medicine takes into account this environment,
which is particularly toxic to children.

Carl Jung wrote: "What most marks the growing child is the
particular affective state that is totally unaware of his parents
and teachers. The hidden misunderstanding between his
parents, secret torments, repressed and concealed desires, all
of this creates in the individual an affective state that slowly
but surely, even if he is unaware of it, finds its way to the
infant soul and engenders the same state in it ... If the adults
are already sensitive to the influences in the environment, we
can predict that the same will be true, in greater proportion,
of the child, whose spirit is still as soft and malleable as wax."

CHAPTER THREE

Applied Social Pediatrics: An Overview

Young people aren't naturally selfish, any more than old folks are naturally wise. Your age doesn't have anything to do with whether you're sensitive or shallow, it's a question of the path your life takes. I can't remember where, but not long ago I read an American Indian saying that goes, "Don't judge a man until you've walked three moons in his moccasins." ... Seen from without, many people's lives seem erroneous, irrational, deranged. It's easy to misunderstand other people and their relationships if we view them from the outside. Only by looking deeper, only by walking three moons in their moccasins can we comprehend their motives, their feelings, what makes them act one way and not another. Understanding comes from humility, not from the pride of knowledge.

Susanna Tamaro, *Follow Your Heart*

Social pediatrics is an approach that brings together the major figures in the child's life to gain a better understanding of the issues and values that are important to each person, with the goal of determining effective action to be taken concerning the child. To find the pathway that will help a child or family, the health-care professional needs to have the ability to seek, discover, and do what needs to be done. While this could be described as an ideal or a mission, the words don't really matter. The essential point is that the helper must be motivated to support a human being who already possesses some personal baggage – feelings, a culture, beliefs, hurts, and dreams – taking care to do no harm.

From the social pediatrics point of view, the professional's role is not limited to offering a product or program or encouraging the child to follow rules or restricted concepts. Instead, the professional's role is to serve as a guide and reference person at a given time and in a given place so that the child and the family can act for themselves – for their own well-being. The entire process is oriented to that little light that animates each person, and all the professional's actions are designed to rekindle the light and keep it burning. To set the process in motion, to understand and support the child, what the professional needs first and foremost is unfailing motivation, solid as a rock.

To understand a child who is suffering or a family in distress and give them the service they need, some fundamental concepts apply. But concepts are not enough – and they may not help at all – unless they are modulated by an approach that features a great deal of empathy, respect, and patience, which will bring about a process of rapprochement and sharing between individuals. This communication process helps us get to know the person, providing a point of reference to his or her anchors and attachments, and, if needed, a change in direction towards those reference points and the person's ability to act. This concept is what we call *empowerment.*

The principle of horizontal intercommunication (see Figure 1) between caregiver and patient is crucial in supporting the person in order to prevent or treat complex problems. This is the only way not only to understand what is going on but, more importantly, to establish an exchange of resources and powers from both sides. This happy mixture of knowledge and experience may be helpful in finding sustainable, child-centred solutions. Overall medical practice leaves no room for a vertical-communication relationship in which the caregiver acts with authority by virtue of his or her knowledge

Figure 1
Horizontal Intercommunication Process

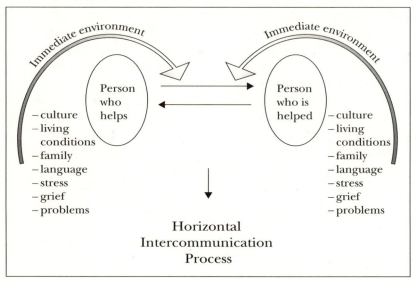

and the patient is subject to a unique truth that does not reflect his or her own knowledge and reference points. If there is no real sharing of sensitivities and knowledge between the professional and the patient, we can hardly expect the individuals we are trying to help to take charge and assume responsibility for their own health and well-being.

Mutual understanding and sharing of knowledge may make it possible to find a consensus, arrive at solutions that make sense (i.e., coherent solutions), and create a dynamic of change that moves towards adapted solutions. Some forms of knowledge are more fundamental than others, specifically the concepts of the parent-child relationship and attachment. First of all, we must arrive at a clear common understanding of the roles that society, the family, and the community should play. Similarly, since certain strategies appear to be more relevant than others, it is helpful to share these. When helping a child who is having problems, it is important to work with the family circle and set in motion the informal networks of the child and family to achieve sustained action. These ways of doing things are in fact based on the so-called "community" and "family" approaches, on which the practice of social pediatrics is based.

HORIZONTAL INTERCOMMUNICATIONS

The Role of Society

A just and supportive society is essential if we hope to be able to meet the needs of children and families. This is the cornerstone that provides the opportunity for optimal development, based on a high level of motivation, thus enabling us to create positive environments and sustain hope.

Seen from this viewpoint, society represents in broad outline the elements in a community that generate a connecting thread that draws together the beliefs and values reflected in families, which in turn become, in a way, the functional units of society. There is a direct correlation between the development and future of children on the one hand and the condition of society and the family on the other. As Garbarino,[1] an expert on child development, aptly notes, it is not enough for society to ensure the continuity of the species and maintain law and order in order to play its supporting role; society must be just in the full ethical sense of the term. It must also meet three basic conditions by offering a historical and cultural framework, providing social coherence, and demonstrating moral legitimacy.

Historical and Cultural Framework

Society conveys the values, beliefs, and traditions that provide a structural base for individuals and give them the system of reference points they need to develop and evolve. The historical framework lends "legitimacy" to children and their families not only by showing them their sources and roots but also by serving as the essential ingredient in the identity process.

The migration of families and individuals, whether it takes place under traumatic circumstances such as political conflict, war, or ethnic clashes, or within the framework of a change process linked to economic, situational, or social problems, sheds light on the important role the historical foundation plays in ensuring the coherence and continuity of personal identity. Stories of young people cut off from their history – immigrants who revolt against their people or their elders, or young natives deprived of their roots – illustrate the usefulness of having such a structural foundation, especially in times of stress and upheaval. Without it the individual is vulnerable and exposed to many risks and destructive responses to trauma, such as alcohol, drugs, delinquency, and criminality.

The concept of culture, strongly linked to the historical perspective and the strength of a society, is another ingredient that promotes the identity and integrity of the individual child. The work of Tobie Nathan, based on clinical experiments with migrant families, reveals the full impact of culture on health and well-being. According to Nathan, it not only makes the social space coherent but also, and most importantly, it makes individuals' interior system coherent, enabling them to enclose their psychic space.[2] The influence of a society's and a family's cultural integrity determines the well-being and development of children in a sort of historical continuity borne by the family. This integrity to some extent justifies the gathering of culturally similar individuals into countries or nations in which they find features that set them apart from other humans. It is important to find your place among those who are close to you culturally in order to assimilate these links, which subsequently make it possible to open up to the outside world and other people. This is no doubt why we naturally enjoy being among those who are like us, and why we are always drawn to the mother country, even after spending many years abroad. Culture is much more than a mask, a colour, or a set of superficial traits. It is an integral part of each individual's dynamic forces, providing structure and impetus. The absence or abandonment of culture leads to blockages and disruptions, which in turn may affect an individual's overall health status.

Social coherence

When a child is born, he has only a physical existence; he has not yet been authorized by the family or recognized by the community. Only by virtue of rites conducted after birth is he integrated into the community of the living.

Mircea Eliade, *The Sacred and the Profane*

The past two decades have not been supportive, to put it mildly, of the cause of families and children – especially not in North America since the heady days of the Baby Boomers. Society and the economy have continued to disintegrate, along with the illusion of supposed prosperity. At the same time, in a highly significant phenomenon, communities have surrendered their supporting role, and families have dispersed – or in many cases, simply split up. Social coherence is an essential ingredient in the structuring of individuals, promoting strong communities that are committed to supporting children and families, and families that feel valued are able to play their pivotal role with their children.

Few would dispute the active role communities must play in supporting children and families and fostering their health and well-being. Our desire to develop healthy communities or towns today goes straight to the heart of the matter. Clearly, communities that are not "healthy" are "sick." A healthy community supports the set of needs associated with the well-being of the individuals who make up that community. More specifically, such a community supports the family units that in turn help form the structural base of individuals.

Social coherence includes feelings of pride and belonging, which promote the autonomy of individuals and pooling of resources. Where social coherence exists, needy families are supported. Children with problems are not deprived of help or just plain excluded – left hungry, out in the cold, neglected, mistreated, or abandoned. To play its role fully, the family absolutely needs a climate of social and economic stability, which fortifies its capacity to support the development of the child.[3]

In a just and coherent society, in a healthy community, the family can exercise its true potential and provide unrestricted support to children. In a just society, the family represents our best hope for the physical, sociocultural, and spiritual integrity of the child.

Moral Legitimacy

The dictionary definition of morality is the science of good and evil. It is also the science of natural laws, the science of purpose, and the ideal order of life. A "moral" society sets forth rules for behaviour, codes for living, and an entire system of ethical values. "Legitimacy" refers to acting in accordance with certain standards that shape daily life and lend meaning to it. We consider it normal to "act properly in society" by following laws, avoiding abuse, and ensuring the safety and well-being of all citizens. The underlying concepts of justice and fairness give meaning to "acting properly." Building on such a moral base, a society develops legislation to prevent evil or protect individuals, and to provide a framework for behaviour, to some extent at least.

In Canada, federal and provincial legislation, such as the new Youth Criminal Justice Act (federal legislation passed in 2002, replacing the Young Offenders Act) and the Youth Protection Act (Quebec legislation passed in 1977) reflects a moral society that has developed a framework for overseeing family practices and the behaviour of young people designed to ensure the best interests of the child. These laws stand as sterling examples of moral legitimacy.

No matter how "moral" a society may be, however, it must never set aside the ethical and spiritual values on which its legitimacy is based, which are designed to provide a framework for the best interests of the child.

No judgment deserves to be called "ethical" that fails to reflect the meaning of acts, and claims to give priority to their supposed reliability over their necessary humanity, that denies emotion, the link between unlinkable things.

Paul Valéry

THE ROLE OF THE FAMILY

The family is indisputably at the heart of the child's development, vouching for the child's well-being. By definition, the family is the central repository of experience, values, and wellness tools for its members, especially the youngest members of the family. As a direct link with the society of which it is the functional unit, the family is the repository for the basic buildings block of development. Intervening with families allows us to have an impact on the primary influence that shapes children's overall integrity and health – in the physical, social, emotional, and spiritual dimensions. The family's global health equation, from which are derived know-how, positive attitudes, and behaviours, is directly linked to the child's global health equation.

Within families, the tasks involved in childcare traditionally fall into two recognized categories.[4] The first category includes material support, training, and supervision – the essential materials of physical integrity and security, such as food, clothing, shelter, hygiene, health care, education, and so on. The second category includes support for cognitive and affective functions, such as socioemotional support (love, esteem, communication, self-actualization, friendship, and values), the education and skills needed for personal development and coping with the stresses of life.

We could add another, less formal dimension to the family's role, one that transcends the parental function. It is connected with the species and the culture, and it involves the underpinnings for the individual, passed down through the generations and through spirituality. This more abstract dimension serves as a foundation for each child's spirit, with the family acting as mediator. In addition to the instrumental functions of an affective or cognitive nature, which are more sensitive to outside intervention, it is an immutable and essential function for the harmonious development of the child.

All these functions of the family help support the child's health and development.[5] The instrumental functions can, if necessary, be supported by various groups or institutions, such as food banks, social housing, and basic health-care services. The affective and cognitive functions can be filled through partnerships within the family circle, by friends, neighbours, and the school. The "superior" functions are inherent to the family in a subconscious way. The only way to transmit the baggage that is so essential to the child is through a harmonious interaction between parent and child.

The Parent-Child Relationship

Parents are the most significant people in a child's life, the people who are able to assume all the roles that are essential to the child's development. Most of all, parents are accustomed to creating the deep links that give meaning to what we call the parent-child relationship and the attachment relationship. The "parents" are, more often than not, those who have a direct biological link to the child, but others may play the parental role in a satisfactory way. They may come from the extended family – aunts, uncles, brothers, sisters, grandparents – or from the family circle or the community, or they may be designated by society, as in the case of foster families. The important thing is that loving people agree to take full and complete charge of children who cannot, for the time being, take care of themselves and steer the children through to adulthood with all the necessary tools for their well-being.

The *parent-child relationship* becomes the instrument that enables the parent to play his or her role to the fullest extent. This unique and delicate exchange between individuals who have already experienced deep links, in most cases, is based on the experiences and life of an adult supporting a developing child, who also has a clearly identified personality and potential. The entire question of continuity and filiation is expressed in this relationship.

Parents are unique individuals who proceed from their own development and their own life experience. In parallel, the child's development is influenced by other factors, such as biology, gender, culture, personal experience, and cultural baggage.[6] Development is a continuous and complex process, and we each have our own image of the process to enable us to understand it. It could be visualized as a *trajectory* (a concept I will discuss in further detail below), fuelled by a set of influencing factors, and evolving over time. A healthy parent-child relationship is a tremendous advantage throughout the trajectory, providing impetus for development. It can even protect the child from negative factors that could be harmful. By all indications, a healthy parent-child relationship ensures that the child develops in a harmonious and long-lasting way. But that relationship is not simple: under the best conditions, it is established in the very first moments of life, and probably well before. It is therefore the result of multiple influences and may undergo perverse effects along the way.[7] The parent-child relationship is essential, but fragile and vulnerable. Everything possible must be done to protect and sustain it. And that is where social pediatrics comes in.

Bigner lists four important characteristics of the parent-child relationship:

1 The relationship corresponds to a social system of two-way communication between an adult and a child;
2 It is subject to ambiguities or questions on the goals and expectations of parenting due to the rapid pace of social change the parents experience;
3 The adult's reasons and motivations for becoming a parent are varied and influence his or her quality of parenting;

4 Being a parent is also a process of development that, by its very nature, is modulated by personal changes and is changed and defined over time. Being a parent thus involves a continuous adaptation process.[8]

Communication between any two individuals is never easy – especially communication that lasts an entire lifetime, in which one of the parties exercises parental authority while the other is in a position of extreme vulnerability. Like any other form of human communication, the parent-child communication system must adapt to different personalities in a mode of mutual understanding and coherence. Since the only thing that can bring about the desired communication is love between parent and child, we must make sure that this love can be expressed freely and on a solid foundation.

Parents are subject to many different irritants in the performance of their duties; the most serious irritants doubtless involve adapting to swift social change and the type of social support they can expect to receive. The role and responsibilities of parents are constantly changing, but the social support that would normally facilitate the parental role is doubtless in decline in our society, which directly affects the quality of the parent-child relationship by making parents less available to their children. For example, parents who work long hours "to make ends meet" deprive themselves of precious contact with their child. They are frequently obliged to give the child to others to look after – that is, when they don't take diversionary tactics such as corralling the child in front of the TV or Nintendo. Other parents, the social outcasts whose numbers are growing, live under minimal conditions for survival, trying to feed their families or put a roof over their heads. These are hardly ideal conditions for parenting or for setting an example of pride and happiness for children to follow.

Being a parent requires having sufficient motivation and maturity to oversee the conditions that promote the child's long-term, balanced development. Being a parent is also a strong emotional experience that unleashes all sorts of reactions and frequently pushes back the boundaries of what is "human." A great deal is expected of a parent – sometimes too much for one person. While there are some very special and extraordinary moments, there are also many times when it all seems too much and parents feel "at the end of their rope." It is precisely at such times that the support system should come into play, immediately and respectfully.

Parents have to show steadfastness, consistency, and most of all, love – three attributes that will inevitably influence the quality of the parent-child relationship. In our practice, parents often confess their fear of being unable to fill the role of parent properly, sometimes for short periods and sometimes for longer. Love is not usually what's lacking at such difficult times – more often than not, it is steadfastness or consistency.

At the root of parents' difficulties, all sorts of problems surface, related to previous experience or circumstances. These may include not having had a significant parental role model when they were young, physical or moral exhaustion in the face of the arduous task of parenting, poor living conditions or persistent poverty, or serious personal problems. Events, incidents, and accidents can influence people in profound ways and modulate parenting abilities as a result, affecting the quality of the parent-child relationship. In every life there are happy events and times of sadness that can either cement or jeopardize that relationship, depending on the personal abilities, motivation, and maturity of the parents and the support they can rely on.

The process of building the parent-child relationship is extremely dynamic. There are high points and low points, but in general the high points prevail. Even in times of adversity, some way can be found to support the child as long as certain conditions are present, especially the unconditional love that parents alone can bring. Confidence is another important condition.

Three constants emerge throughout the process. First of all, the parent is a human being with needs and hopes who is subject to change. Parents generally embark on the parent-child relationship with confidence and in good faith, sometimes somewhat naively, with the feeling that they are not alone in the task and will not be alone in the future. The decision is personal, but it is based on a consensus with the community and society.

The second constant is society's universal commitment to maintaining conditions that are conducive to both child and parent so that a healthy relationship is established between them and continues – the relationship that is so essential to the full development of the child. Under such conditions, when a problem arises, an unhappy event such as divorce occurs, or there is some change in living conditions, the community should be prepared to intervene, provide support, and make things easier. There is no question here of taking the place of the family – simply lending a hand at the right time and in the right way to let the family become whole again and stay together.

The third constant, one that we must never lose sight of, is the fact that in the child's eyes what counts is the security of the relationship with the parent and being clear on the changes they are going through. The child must be able to count on the parent at all times; if that is not possible, the parent must give the child permission to count on someone else for a set period of time in order to preserve the child's sense of security and attachment to the parent. The child must also be able to understand the changes and be given a clear explanation in age-appropriate terms. The child must understand the reasons for a break-up, for example, and be told that it is not his or her fault. The child should be spared the anguish of having to cope with too many changes at once; above all, in times of trouble a child should have someone close on hand – a parent, teacher, social worker, or whomever the child has chosen in full confidence. In this

way the foundation of a healthy relationship will be pre-
served even if it must be fragmented temporarily.

Being a good parent, even in a time of crisis, means understanding what the child needs and taking the necessary steps
to safeguard the consistency of the relationship, which is so
important to the child's development. Being a good parent
provides an opportunity to serve as a positive, secure role
model – the prime determinant in the child's optimal development. Being a loving and supportive parent provides the
opportunity to protect the child from negative environments
that can jeopardize a child's well-being.[9]

Attachment: The Strongest Link

Attachment expresses the parent-child relationship at its
best. It is a total and long-lasting connection that serves as
the foundation for personal development throughout life.
The more complete and harmonious the attachment, the
more solid – even indestructible – the foundation will be.

Bowlby and Ainsworth, two well-known authors in this
field, conducted in-depth research on attachment and the essential role it plays in child development.[10] Hence the *theory
of attachment,* which dictates that the deep emotional connection between child and parent promotes the child's sense of
confidence and competence. Attachment has even been said
to be the only way for a child to survive. Attachment affects
the quality of the parent-child relationship in the long term –
in fact, for life.[11]

The nature of attachment and its effects vary with age and are
manifested in different ways at different stages of development.
In the first few months or years, attachment is what allows a child
to explore and get to know the world. Later on, it continues to
serve as a foundation and reference point for progress in life. As
Bowlby states, "It endures over time and space."[12]

Attachment is defined both as a mode of parent-child interrelation that can set the child's global development in motion in a

coherent and persistent way, and as the child's connection with the environment.[13] It also serves as a system that regulates the parent-child relationship, based on a welcoming attitude, confidence, security, availability, consistency, motivation and love. Attachment applies to all humans universally. It is also observed in the animal world, as various experimental studies have shown. Attachment promotes the child's development, as well as several other factors, such as the stability of environments and personal characteristics of a biological, historical, or cultural nature. But attachment clearly remains the principal factor.

Attachment is reflected in the sensitivity to signals that exists between child and parents, as shown by gestures, sounds, and looks. It also reveals the motivations of the parties involved. It is shown through a wide range of attitudes and behaviours, in various modes and contexts. The personality of the child and parents, their previous experience, current stage of life and development, as well as contexts and culture, influence the expression of attachment. In some people, it will be extremely *concrete*, taking the form of physical contact, words, and intense looks in response to needs shown by the child or by the parent. In other people at other times, attachment will be more discreet, more "interior," expressed by the juxtaposition of objects or people. But the true essence of attachment will always be the same and the ingredients consistent, based on empathy, comforting, presence, permanence, and being available to the other person.

As an illustration, let's examine the rites by which various societies, such as traditional aboriginal communities, welcome a child into the world. These rites involve welcoming and identifying the child at birth or at certain times of life. The goal is to signify to the community at large the importance of establishing a solid attachment. It is also a way of telling the child and the parents in no uncertain terms that a high degree of importance is attached to the child and that this new being "belongs" in a non-exclusive way. This sends a concrete signal that the community approves of and is taking charge of the child alongside the parents. It is the beginning of a true foundation that gives the whole family a sense of security and serves as an extremely strong motivating factor.

Since attachment is a durable manifestation of parental competence and influence, it gives the child means of support that will last through the developmental stage and remain useful tools even in adult life. Parents, and others who have a capacity for attachment, will serve as *facilitators* to structure the child's personality, transmit cultural understanding of the social structure, and guide the child's various interactions with his or her environment. Attachment, which creates a sense of *security* since it is based on unfailing confidence, provides sufficient representation of reality by making the world predictable, and thus less menacing. This helps the child deal with the world and provides a base of self-esteem for life. Through attachment, the parent also plays the role of *interpreter* of certain traumatic events, such as major crises, grieving, emotional hurts, and ill treatment. It serves as a tool for solving most of the problems the child will have to deal with during childhood and adolescence.

Attachment is essential to developing the integrative mechanisms that will help the child to develop and adapt – and to survive. A child who has acquired the regulatory mechanisms provided by attachment will be able to face up to adversity more easily, or cope with various forms of stress that can occur at any time. A child who has this foundation and is the victim of mistreatment at some point can use the foundation as a reference point and be better protected against the traumatic event, as his or her internal representation of the event will be less disturbing and more rational. The suffering will be just as great, but the consequences and the scars will doubtless be less serious. The child might say to himself, "Daddy didn't beat me because I'm bad, he was just tired ..."

This way of integrating serious problems gives children an easier way out when problems arise. It may even help them to avoid despair, which not only impedes development but can lead to major traumas, including delinquency, drug abuse, or even suicide.

The Clinical Theory of Attachment

Attachment theory is extremely useful in the clinic. It is possible to evaluate the presence or absence of attachment between parent and child based on certain scientifically defined criteria.[14] This information is extremely valuable in understanding a child's development problems or disorders. Essentially, it provides reasons for certain problems and makes it easier to plan what to do with the child and the parents. The presence of secure attachment is shown by:

- frequent affectionate exchanges between parent and child;
- the tendency to seek comfort from a parent when the child is afraid or frustrated;
- certainty that the parent will help;
- a child's referring to the parent for approval or permission;
- the quality of the relationship during or after a separation.

These are some of the indicators that can help professionals observing the parent-child interrelation to form a useful clinical opinion.

Attachment is one of the important strengths the child can count on in times of trouble. It also represents a major protective factor that ensures the child's harmonious development.

THE CONCEPT OF PARTNERSHIP

When it comes to medical care for children, the partnership between parents and health-care professionals does not have a long history. It was only about 20 years ago that the concept of a partnership involving all the major parties emerged, and its application is still, unfortunately, limited. However, we are now discovering the full impact of parent participation on the effects of measures taken to ensure children's health and well-being.

The concept has really only come to the fore since the World Health Organization's Alma Alta Declaration of 1978,[15] which implicitly stated that everyone has the right to participate individually and collectively in the promotion and protection of his or her health. The partnership concept was reinforced by the United Nations Convention on the Rights of the Child, which recognizes children's rights in the context of parents' rights and responsibilities. Article 18 recognizes the parents' primary responsibility for the care of the child, and society's duty to help them fulfill that responsibility.[16]

Despite the fact that experience in various domains of health care and education has shown the usefulness of having parents play an active role in their children's well-being, such participation often meets with major resistance due to the dominating attitude of certain institutions or professions, which still believe that they are the only ones who can deal with children's problems and make the appropriate decisions on their behalf.

The concept of teaming up with the parents essentially means a joint involvement in what will be done for the children by sharing the highly professional view of health care or well-being on the one hand and the more pragmatic view of the parent on the other. While getting parents involved means sharing knowledge, techniques, and skills, the most important part is developing a respectful relationship of support, based on parents' strengths, so that they can make the right decisions for their child.[17] Instead of a more domineering model of association, this partnership model is based on recognition, sharing, negotiation, and accountability. By its very nature, it recognizes the crucial role of the parents, supporting and sustaining them in that role.

Partnership with parents is a rather specialized approach that is not yet widely used – primarily because it involves an egalitarian exchange and a certain loss of direct power over professional interventions. As a result, it requires a major shift in habits and practices on the part of most professionals. The approach is an attractive one, however: sharing powers

actually gives both parties more power when it comes to preventing illness, supporting individuals, and improving children's living conditions, with greater repercussions for their
health and well-being. With proper support, the person in
charge, who is certainly the most credible and most closely involved with the child, becomes the best promoter of the
child's health.

The Partnership Approach

The partnership approach can be applied at different levels:
between the parent and the professional, by multidisciplinary or community groups, or through the parent's direct
participation in making decisions and planning what treatments and services the child will receive. The partnership approach recognizes the parent's essential and unique role in
order to ensure children's well-being by placing them at the
centre of decisions and procedures. This type of partnership
includes the parent in an egalitarian, respectful, dynamic,
and responsible relationship designed to meet the child's
various needs. Even parents who are facing personal problems, whether through a lack of knowledge of how to parent
or because they have themselves experienced trauma or
stress, and are having difficulty doing their job as parents can
benefit from a partnership approach that includes them,
with all their strengths and weaknesses.

In the case of abusive or negligent parents, a partnership
approach that involve the parents is much more likely to succeed than excluding them in a punitive or authoritarian
model. It becomes possible to work directly on the root
causes of the problem based on an integrated-approach
model in which all factors are taken into consideration to arrive at a solution that is adapted to meet the child's needs. If
the parent's condition requires therapy, the health-care professional can make the appropriate arrangements. If the
child requires protection, that can be arranged with the

agreement of the parent in charge. If the parties request a period of respite, the system can make sure that they get one.

To work with the parents and allow them to play their full role, as we have seen, it is a good idea to share both knowledge and power, to respect the parents' beliefs and experiences (i.e., their culture), and to negotiate ideas and procedures based on the child's needs. In this spirit, the first step is to get to know the parents and the family, meeting them in a place where everyone is comfortable – if necessary, on their home turf or in a neutral setting where everyone feels free to express their expectations. During this initial meeting the professional will start to gain acceptance and assess the strengths and weaknesses of the family, both parents and child, not just draw up a negative list of problems. Those strengths will emerge from the exchange as questions are asked in a nonjudgmental way, premised on a clear understanding of the objective – the best interests of the child. The professional is not an inquisitor, but he or she does need to obtain some accurate information in order to have a complete picture of the situation in which the child lives so that a plan can be drawn up based on a full understanding.

The professional's next job is to perform a quick assessment of the parents' strengths and weaknesses, with the aim of putting the strengths to work and counterbalancing the weaknesses on a continuum of steps designed to ensure the child's well-being. Bear in mind that parents usually have some child-raising skills, but they are frequently concealed by events and difficult living conditions. Sometimes simply giving the parent "permission" to act is enough to discover unsuspected strengths and skills.

Observing the attitudes of and interactions between parent and child during the interview will elicit a goldmine of important information on habits and emotions, as well as factors that can affect the child's health or underlying reasons for certain problems. Observation will also raise various questions on the parents' perception and expectations of the child, how the parents assess themselves, and whether they are willing to make certain changes and become more involved or differently involved in helping the child. At this stage, affinities are formed and a shared interest in taking steps to help the child emerges. This is what is really at stake in the partnership.

Parents' Strengths

To help us understand what we're looking for in terms of parents' strengths, here are some key characteristics, as cited by Green:[18]

- The parent considers health a priority.
- The parent has fun with the child.
- The parent recognizes signals from and needs of the child and responds in a satisfactory way.
- The parent offers the child emotional support and reassurance as needed and protects the child from overwhelming stress.
- The parent encourages and congratulates the child and stimulates the child's self-esteem.
- The parent has a warm attitude and communicates with ease.
- The parent is healthy in mind and body (personal abilities).
- The parent has an extended mutual support network.
- The parent teaches the child healthy habits.
- The parent encourages independence, maturity, and success.
- The parent is a positive role model.

These qualities are important tools that enable a parent to influence the child's development in a positive trajectory, and the presence of such strengths creates a favourable environment. It is important to remember, however, that ways and means of acting to create such a favourable environment vary from family to family and from culture to culture. We must judge by the end result, not only by ways of doing things – which makes it all the more important to have fruitful exchanges and negotiation. It is also important to recognize the limitations of having parents and families participate, based on their own characteristics or the extent to which they are currently available. Finally, we must act prudently and not expect too much of some parents, adapting their role accordingly.

Types of Partnerships

Based on their experiences in the medical field, researchers Doherty and Baird[19] have developed a model that establishes parents' level of commitment and possible types of partnerships. The model is useful for evaluating the current level of commitment and the family's potential commitment in the future. It can also be used in working with the parent to draw up a joint action plan that will reflect the expectations and abilities of each party with a view to maximum effectiveness. The model is based on four levels of commitment.

Level 1 involves mainly the traditional aspects of professional practice, in which the professional-family exchange takes place on the cognitive level and is a one-way street. This is the biomedical model, which places the accent on practical or medical/legal aspects associated with the illness, and in which communication plays a small role or none at all.

Level 2 involves a more concrete mode of cooperation between the professional and the family, but this is still limited to motivations behind the precise diagnosis and follow-up treatment. At this level, the parent still serves only as an information source and the person who carries out the treatment.

Level 3 puts the accent on the emotional factors and stresses involved in the genesis of the problems and illnesses. The sharing and exchange of information begin at this level, significantly broadening the communication field. Parents are no longer participating purely as an accessory. Their participation is now part of the dynamic for the child's health and well-being.

Level 4 is where the entire family system enters the picture. Everyone is asked to participate in understanding the child's problems, taking preventive and curative action, and generally getting involved with the child. This intervention may take place during family meetings, at which certain habits, attitudes, or beliefs are reviewed according to an explanatory symptom-based model. A true partnership involving responsibility for identified needs is emerging at this point. This level also provides an opportunity to discuss the set of factors that are jeopardizing the child's health and factors that could protect or improve the child's general well-being. Beyond purely medical considerations, all the elements that affect the global environment, such as financial problems, mental disorders, marital discord, and family violence, are now taken into consideration. The professional can adopt or create diversified and adapted communication tools at this stage, and most importantly, can also develop an important support network for the child.

The Prevention Circle

To take the partnership concept a little farther, let's look at some innovative concepts that have been tested in specific real-life settings. For example, a professional's openness to parent participation could lead to another, much more advanced form of partnership: *the prevention circle*. This concept originated in the highly meaningful circle that aboriginals hold dear. Traditionally, the circle would be called upon to share ideas and solve all sorts of problems that involved the community, based on the principles of common strengths and mutual confidence. More recently, it has been used in the form of *justice circles* to commit the community and victims to the rehabilitation of criminals. To the best of my knowledge, it has not yet been used in everyday life to solve children's problems or prevent situations that could be dangerous for them.

The idea of having *prevention circles* in the family and in the network can sometimes help decode problem behaviours or specific problems children and teens are having. This approach is based on global health concepts and the importance of environment in personal development, especially for children. The essential point is to share knowledge, experience, explanations, and solutions with the parties involved and with those who have an interest in the child's well-being, in order to arrive at a consensus in which those present, or at least some of them, make a commitment to the best interests of the child.

This approach can be applied in various ways, as long as the basic concept is adhered to and a meeting is set up at which information is shared and those with an interest in the child's well-being make a commitment. This may simply involve the child's parents, friends, neighbours, and professionals sitting around the kitchen table. Or the meeting may bring the parents and the child together with various professionals from different fields or even different cultures to come up with some statements they can agree on, share some hypotheses, and arrive at a consensus on what further steps should be taken. In my experience, the prevention-circle approach has frequently proven to be an effective method of changing difficult trajectories, refocusing the identity of troubled teens, such as high-school dropouts, helping to foster a more secure attachment, or preventing more serious problems.

From a more rational standpoint, the idea of the prevention circle may seem "magical," but this gathering of knowledge and energy frequently generates unexpected results that are most desirable for the child. The method, which requires rather intense participation by the primary professional, is not for everyone; but in any major intervention with a child, it is worth considering a certain form of contract with parents and families. The advantage of such an agreement is that expectations are clearly stated, and most of all, each party's roles and mandates are spelled out from the standpoint of mutual commitment, which is conducive to finding customized solutions. "The hallmark of a family-oriented physician will be that he or she will make the option of assembling the family a routine part of the therapeutic contract for a number of serious or chronic problems, traditional biomedical problems as well as explicitly psychosocial problems."[20]

THE NETWORK: A GLOBAL APPROACH

Keeping children healthy and supporting their development requires a global approach. This involves making links with the networks that surround the child to ensure that the required steps are taken in the most effective way and that continuity is maintained.

In 1991, a Quebec government task force on youth suggested that "extremely early intervention in children's lives is the best way to invest in the creation of contexts that can set children on the right road as young as possible, so that affection, success, and a sense of identify and self-confidence become the best protective tools. We need to invest in improving children's living places (family, school, daycare, and neighbourhood) if we want them to develop the skills that will keep them [from needing] health care and rehabilitation services."[21]

A global approach considers all the factors and catalysts and the many facets of a problem in order to take effective action with a child or group of children. To explain and understand the child's health problems and properly define what actions should be taken and what pathways should be followed, it is always a good idea to consult the networks that surround the child and get them involved. These would include the networks of parents, friends, neighbours and other contacts, the school, recreation centre, even people on the street at times. All of these networks matter, since they all have a connection with the child and can influence him or her directly.

A network is by definition a system or chain with many interconnections or interrelations. Every child has a network and no child is an island. The child is surrounded by various influences – from parents, the extended family, and the community. The network includes a vast range of influences, but it is also what partially defines the child's identity and has an ongoing impact on how the child develops. To return to Tobie Nathan's image, this is the context of the text, or the background of the subject we are considering. The child is not a laboratory animal who can be rooted out of his milieu to be probed or protected, because the child's life is exactly that – his milieu. In fact, solutions to most children's problems lie within those milieux – hence the importance of hooking up with those networks.

This approach enables us to have an impact on the child's network of influences in a direct and deep way by attempting to establish or reconstitute a state of balance with the child and relying on the intrinsic forces of each individual. The network approach, which reflects and involves the child's environments, also includes the concepts of community participation and multidisciplinary and intersectorial approaches. It is also based on the principles of the family approach. It takes place on a local level, under the child's own living conditions, and according to the accepted rules and customs of that milieu.

The importance of community participation was clearly stated in 1978 at the Alma Ata Conference, which declared that primary health care should be "made universally accessible to individuals and families in the community through their full participation at a cost that the community and country can afford to maintain at every stage of their development."[22]

Problems That Can be Solved by the Community

Many children's health problems can be presented for examination and community participation, especially multifaceted problems and those with a major social component. This type of problem also requires multifaceted solutions and solutions the family and the community deem to be of great importance. Since these specific problems have great potential for mobilizing the community, the local solutions that are envisioned are generally effective.[23] Conditions that can benefit from this approach include accidents and poisonings, respiratory problems (asthma), dental problems, eating disorders, violence and neglect, school problems, behavioural problems and conduct disorders, affective disorders, developmental difficulties, and other problems. All troubled children with special needs should be able to enjoy the benefits of this approach, as they experience a whole set of problems that jeopardize their health and development, which are generally preventable or can be cured with the active participation of various milieux working together in an integrated way.

Here are three examples of participation models or approaches that can involve the community:

1 *Community participation.* This is a major asset when working with children and teens. According to some experts,[24] it is absolutely indispensable for primary health problems, because it actively involves a group of people from the community in clearly defining needs and objectives, priorities, mobilizing resources, overseeing results, and making the necessary readjustments. Community interven-

tion takes control of the situation to create positive environments. The resulting impact on the child's health is not just cumulative but multiplied many times over.[25]

2 *The multidisciplinary approach.* This involves more commitment by professionals from various disciplines, who *act* together in a concerted way to attain a common goal. With the network approach, the participation of professionals is of primary importance, as it helps give the community certain techniques and tools for expressing their needs and expectations. It also serves to strengthen the community's capacity for effective action. However, this can be a delicate operation since the subtext, in terms of local action, is a major adjustment in roles and power sharing. The multidisciplinary system rules out any hierarchical relationship between caregiver and patient in which the former exerts total authority and the latter passively follows recommendations and treatments. For health-care professionals, it involves sharing values and knowledge with the community that will improve the steps that are eventually taken for the community. Here, control lies in the hands not of the professionals but of the community, which will take action in the best interests of the child in light of the consensus arrived at by all the players.

One example is perinatal programs. In Quebec, the program known as Naître égaux et grandir en santé[26] (Born Equal, Growing up Healthy) shows the interest aroused by a network approach with community participation. The consensus of committed health-care professionals in the program is fundamental to its success. Everyone has a clear role to play, which is established with a local professional who is responsible for communicating adapted information to individuals and helping them meet their needs, while respecting the common objective of improving the child's state of health and well-being. A precise goal, a consensus for action and community mobilization – it all adds up when it comes to caring for children.

3 *The intersectoral approach* involves activating mutual support systems in the child's and the family's environment that have an interrelated effect on the child's health and well-being. Children do not live in isolation in their families. Their environment is made up of multiple support systems that extend well beyond the health-care and social-service network, including relatives and friends, local and national policies, the state of the economy, access to education, the quality of legislation, and the values held by society.[27] These systems are the basis for a broader, intersectoral action that enriches the network approach (see Figure 2).

Developing a Network

The *network* is a complex and extremely dynamic concept. Building a network requires the participation of the community, interested professionals, and people from influential sectors, all taking action for the well-being of children. Villes en santé and Écoles en santé [Healthy Towns and Healthy Schools], two health-promotion projects developed in Quebec, illustrate the network approach to promoting child health. The projects are designed to mobilize a group of partners to influence public health-care policy, create supportive environments, decide on local actions to be taken, and give new hope to children by changing their health-care trajectory. The network approach then becomes a broad-based intervention by many people, sometimes the whole community, influencing determinants and causes of health and well-being. It also becomes an essential prerequisite for promoting the health of children and families.

The network approach can also be used to solve specific problems children face, such as dropping out of school, teenage pregnancy, the risk of suicide, and delinquency. Solutions to these problems, which have multiple causes and serious consequences for society, can only be found through a collective effort to work with children to develop a range of

Figure 2
Targets and Strategies for Child Health Promotion

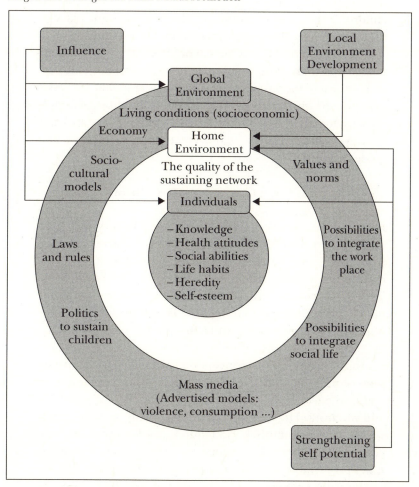

Source: Guide de formation « Développement d'un programme concerté dans un contexte multisectoriel: Promotion de la santé et prévention primaire des toxicomanies chez les jeunes, » *module 4, Service de formation-réseau,* MSSS, 1992.

measures that can be taken before problems arise, working on factors and causes during the most sensitive times in children's lives. Action must be taken in the right place at the right time, with the individuals who are most involved.

Whether the problem is mental or physical, the network approach can make a difference. Common sense and many examples bear witness to the preventive or therapeutic successes experienced with troubled children when a number of people working together, based on a variety of experiences and allegiances, come together in the community to support and guide children.

THE CHILD'S TRAJECTORY

Every person and every event has a natural history, with a beginning and an end. The *trajectory* is what takes a person from the beginning to the end – the trajectory of life, from conception to birth, childhood, adolescence, and adulthood. What concerns us here, of course, is the trajectory of childhood, which we hope to influence. That trajectory has some important characteristics, which are often impossible to predict.

From the moment of conception the child is in a constant state of motion, and that level of physical development only picks up pace. Moods and emotions – everything is moving and vibrating. The trip along the trajectory is made in stages, which involve ambushes and failures as well as wins and successes. The process is dynamic and observable; it is sometimes predictable and can frequently be influenced.

The child's trajectory is partly determined by the genetic and cultural factors that shape part of his or her body and soul, but along the way a set of influential factors comes into play, the result of living conditions and habits, the global environment, and sheer chance. These factors colour the child's life, either placing the child at risk or providing protection.

The child's development trajectory is based on a series of acquisitions of various kinds and levels of maturity in physical, intellectual, social, and emotional terms. It consists of wins and losses, successes and failures, joy and sadness. Along the way, alliances are formed, models developed, and strengths aquired. This trajectory defines the child's self-esteem, confidence, and security. All this work is constantly modulated by a base of attachment to significant figures who serve as a foundation and reference point. The more solid and secure the base, the greater the child's capacity to cope with failure or sadness, since the child can dig deep for new energies, ensuring a positive trajectory. The more fragile and poorly anchored the base, the weaker the child's abilities and the more fragile the development trajectory will become.

In the clinic, the concept of the child's trajectory is useful because it gives professionals a tool to use in observing the child, accompanying him or her if needed, giving the child a solid base, and most of all, being present at the right time in the right way. Careful observation can reveal the precursors of problems or catastrophes, even unusual attitudes or behaviours. Certain dangers that arise can be offset by acting quickly. Risks and alarm signals may be related to the child, and to his or her temperament, experiences, and living habits. They may originate in the child's environment, family, school, friends, the sociocultural environment, or economic conditions; they may even be due to lack of access to quality services. The trajectory concept makes it possible to enter the child's dynamic for change and have a positive influence on the final result.

Studies by psychologist Richard Tremblay[28] provide persuasive evidence of the dynamic of the child's trajectory and the importance of acting quickly as soon as signs are observed that may impede a satisfactory trajectory. Intervention is indicated as soon as a young child in daycare shows signs of aggressive behaviour towards peers, for instance. In fact, the risk of having behavioural problems or conduct disorders is

Figure 3
Structuring Base: Attachment, Identity, Affiliation, Culture

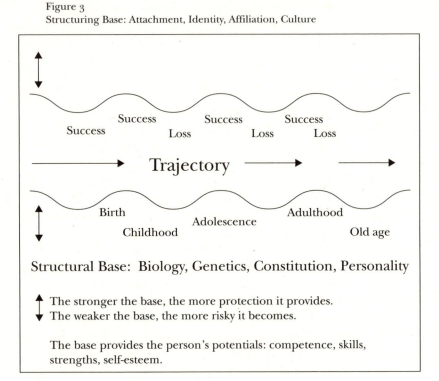

Structural Base: Biology, Genetics, Constitution, Personality

The stronger the base, the more protection it provides.
The weaker the base, the more risky it becomes.

The base provides the person's potentials: competence, skills,
strengths, self-esteem.

greater in these children once they reach school age. If interventions are properly managed and take place at an early
stage, there is reason to believe that such problems can be
avoided later on.

Figure 3 shows the child's trajectory, including successes
and setbacks, at various stages of life. The trajectory rests on
two kinds of foundations: the formative foundation refers to
attachment to significant individuals, identity and culture,
while the structural foundation shows what modulates the
evolution of the trajectory: biological and genetic acquisitions, the child's constitutional inheritance, and personality.

Figure 4 illustrates the dynamic of the trajectory concept
as part of a global community approach in a network.

Figure 4
Child's Trajectory at School – Possible Interventions

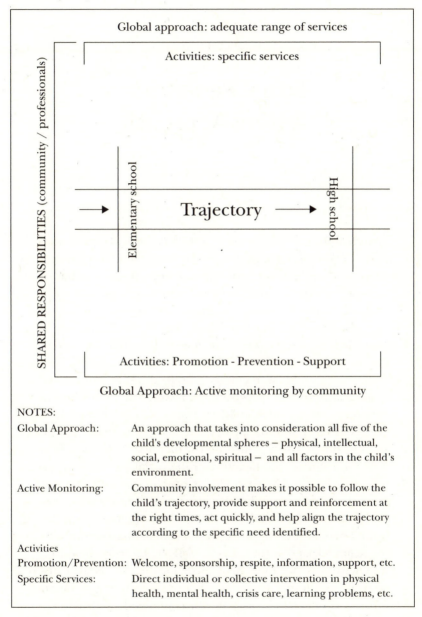

NOTES:

Global Approach:	An approach that takes into consideration all five of the child's developmental spheres – physical, intellectual, social, emotional, spiritual – and all factors in the child's environment.
Active Monitoring:	Community involvement makes it possible to follow the child's trajectory, provide support and reinforcement at the right times, act quickly, and help align the trajectory according to the specific need identified.

Activities
Promotion/Prevention: Welcome, sponsorship, respite, information, support, etc.
Specific Services: Direct individual or collective intervention in physical health, mental health, crisis care, learning problems, etc.

CHAPTER FOUR

Social Pediatrics: A New Approach

CHARACTERISTICS AND APPLICATIONS

The challenges posed by the *United Nations Convention on the Rights of the Child* have led various authors, including B. Lindstrom and N. Spencer,[1] to consider developing a different approach designed to achieve the new objectives of health set forth in the Convention. Since traditional pediatrics has in the past primarily concerned itself with children's diseases, it is now suggested that, due to the complex factors that lie at the root of most children's health problems, a new dimension should be integrated into health care and ways of doing things should be broadened by forming links with the environments in which children live. This does not mean a divorce from traditional pediatrics – rather, it means that we are no longer solely concerned with physical factors. It is time for a shift in the meaning of the social and family contexts that have such harsh effects on children's health and the genesis of illness. What this means is that health-care professionals who treat children should be permitted to go beyond illness in their approach and become more sensitive to the major social determinants that affect children's health.

Pediatrics is the branch of medicine that deals with diseases of children.[2] However, children's health is a much broader concept that takes into account both biopsychosocial issues and extrinsic phenomena – in other words, the whole set of environmental, cultural, emotional, and spiritual influences.

The World Health Organization defines health as not only the absence of illness but an integral state of physical, mental, and social well-being. That definition seems rather incomplete, however, when applied to social pediatrics. In our field other concepts also apply, including ethics in terms of the services we offer, and harmony in terms of children's development. The child's health provides a foundation for developing personal abilities and skills, striving to bring full circle a lifecycle that has a history, an extended duration, and an outcome. It should therefore come as no surprise that *social pediatrics* was born of an ethical concern for the health of children – basically, from the following observation: that in nearly all societies[3] vulnerable and disadvantaged children suffer not only from much higher rates of morbidity and mortality but also from a flagrant diminution of their abilities and their potential for harmonious development. In fact, despite great changes and improvements in the quality of and access to health care in industrialized countries and despite changes over the past few decades in the spectre of diseases and problems that affect children's health, vulnerable children remain the most affected; what's more, they have not benefited from the collective improvement of health status. While concern for justice for all children is hardly new, the level of interest in this cause has risen markedly over the past 20 years. Social pediatrics, though still in its infancy as a discipline, fully supports this philosophy. The practice of social pediatrics targets all children who are vulnerable, involves the assistance of various professionals, and proceeds from a global approach. And it remains deeply committed to justice for children.

In recent years, diseases that could more aptly be called "social" have replaced a number of infectious diseases that have practically disappeared. While technology has taken giant leaps and disease control systems are much more sophisticated, the fact remains that the socioeconomic gradient[4] of disease has remained relatively stable, particularly for children. There are great inequities and large gaps between children from advantaged areas and those from disadvantaged areas in terms of health and illness – in the same country or even the same city. For example, there is often a huge gap between rates of low-birthweight babies in relatively rich and poor neighbourhoods in the same city, with all the related potential complications. In Montreal, the Public Health Department's Born Equal, Growing up Healthy program addresses just this problem. Hence the importance of taking a different approach, one that focuses on environments, working with local people to find solutions that attempt to reduce inequities, especially those that affect childhood. This is still pediatrics – but a more socially engaged type of pediatrics that refers to dramatic population data and works closely with more structured community programs designed to improve the health and well-being of children.

Social pediatrics strives to place children and their health in a more global context that reflects the social, economic, cultural, and political environment. While this is certainly a departure, it has the definite advantage of going straight to the heart of children's health and enlisting the services of a group of professionals with a special interest in their cause. Köhler[5] defines the discipline in terms of three particular levels:

1 Children's health problems with significant social determinants, e.g., poor nutrition of children in impoverished areas;
2 Children's health problems that have social consequences, e.g., dropping out of school, which leads to behavioural problems or difficulty adjusting to the school environment;
3 Children's health care in society, e.g., equity of and access to adapted health-care services, care for disabled children, or for those suffering from chronic diseases.

The practice of social pediatrics places the accent on given populations of children in particular surroundings, such as children from impoverished areas, those with special needs, children who are especially vulnerable, and children who need to be accompanied or protected. This type of practice derives from different levels of knowledge and expertise, borrowing tools and strategies used in public health and community health.

According to Debré,[6] social pediatrics is actually a meeting place and forum for fertile exchanges between a number of disciplines. From public health, social pediatrics borrows techniques that deal with the determinants and consequences of children's health status, improving both prevention and cure. It also borrows from public health various tools used to improve the planning and organization of health-care services adapted to specific populations of children. As noted by Haggerty,[7] in general, eight percent of sick children are actually seen by a physician, two percent are admitted to hospital, and more than sixty percent are cared for exclusively by their mothers. Knowing this should help us plan improved prevention methods that are better adapted to the needs of children. It goes without saying that our priority should be to provide appropriate accessible information to parents to help them give their children better care.

Although social pediatrics intervenes with the child and his or her state of health, the impact is felt on the family and on the community over the short and long terms. It affects the dynamic of families, their interactions in their community, the psychosocial balance, and the organization of services. The practice of social pediatrics borrows from community health and sets itself against a backdrop of primary health care – both preventive and curative. The steps that are taken will be integrated into the community, based on an interdisciplinary and intersectoral model. In this sense, social pediatrics can only be practised if the professionals who are involved function close to the individuals who make up the child's universe and establish relationships with them. "Social" pediatricians must therefore also be "community" pediatricians if they want to mobilize families and communities to provide adequate, extensive, and more accessible care for children.

The objective of social pediatrics is therefore to *give children better and more suitable care,* working with the community. Helping to improve family life and strengthening ties to the community have a positive impact on children's health. Social pediatrics takes an integrated approach to helping populations of needy children – and those needs are specific in the sense that they are frequently nonmedical, of long duration, and primarily social.[8]

A NEW MISSION FOR PEDIATRICIANS

Right from the start and almost by definition, pediatricians are motivated to promote children's health, work for access to basic care, and improve systems for providing curative care. They are frequently active members of the community, ardent defenders of children's rights, and recognized for their influential role in the health and well-being of children. Many pediatricians are involved in research and epidemiology,[9] while others work on projects designed to support children and families or as public health consultants. In Canada, however, the social and community commitment of pediatricians is somewhat fragmented and isolated. The broader role of the social pediatrician remains, unfortunately, marginal.[10]

Pediatricians today must deal with new issues and evolving roles in view of other realities: new morbidities, old diseases that are resurfacing, and health problems arising from globalization and migration. Most of all, they have to face new – or at least newly discovered – problems: children suffering from the consequences of war or grinding poverty, families torn apart or brutally wiped out, and intolerable incidents of violence that are now coming to light. All of these have dramatic effects on children's health and development, and only a broad-based team of individuals and professionals can act effectively in the face of these phenomena. Such a team, deployed on-site, should include everyone who has responsibility for the children in such milieux. The teams will vary according to the place and the circumstances, but they will invariably include responsible and significant individuals, both professionals (physician, social worker, teacher, educator, etc.) and, most importantly, people from the child's milieu (neighbours, caregivers, babysitters, and supervisors). As the direct representatives of the community, through their commitment to and love for the children, they greatly increase the value of whatever measures are taken and make them much more effective. In this sense, the pediatrician or other professional involved can become a unifying force, moderator, and supporter, in the best interests of the child.

The phenomenon of social and family isolation, as well as the growing problem of exclusion, requires a new type of commitment from local partners, professionals from various disciplines, and agents from various sectors.[11] Pediatricians have a key role to play in promoting the child's health and well-being.

Social pediatricians should target the most vulnerable populations of children – those who come from impoverished areas, victimized children, and those with special needs. They must work with the community to develop a new paradigm of care. Influential figures in the child's life must be consulted, actively and as equals, and the child must be seen in his or her context. In a city like Montreal, for example, where there are two major teaching hospitals that treat children, where curative care has attained a high level of excellence, we find in the very shadow of those institutions whole groups of children who are experiencing extreme difficulty on the physical, social, and psychological levels, as well as families experiencing an alarming level of stress. There are whole neighbourhoods of underfed, neglected, or abandoned children living in direst poverty. Families are marginal, and their children are growing up in a world of exclusion and bare survival that is not conducive to their development or quality of life (see Figures 5 and 6).

Figure 5
Mechanism for Exclusion

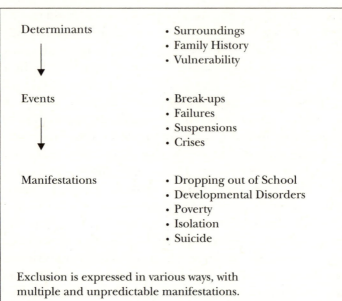

Determinants

- Surroundings
- Family History
- Vulnerability

Events

- Break-ups
- Failures
- Suspensions
- Crises

Manifestations

- Dropping out of School
- Developmental Disorders
- Poverty
- Isolation
- Suicide

Exclusion is expressed in various ways, with
multiple and unpredictable manifestations.

The time has come for pediatricians to speak out. The time has come for pediatricians to refocus their activities on practices that not only relieve illness (which is currently being done quite well) but, above all, create environments conducive to the health of all children. One of the most specific roles of the committed physician will be to improve family life by helping families to develop their own skills and find their own long-lasting solutions. To do this and to adapt[12] to the many and complex needs of children and families, the knowledge and methods to which the physician has access must be continually adapted, redefined, and improved.

Like Haggerty, I believe that such roles as evaluating the risks of new children's health problems and linking up with other professionals to prevent and treat such problems will become an integral part of the pediatrician's job in future – and this dovetails perfectly with the changing needs of children.

Figure 6
Consequences of Exclusion

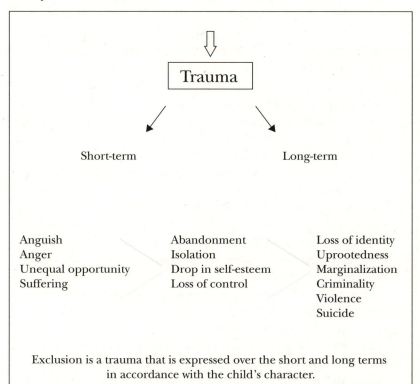

Short-term		Long-term
Anguish	Abandonment	Loss of identity
Anger	Isolation	Uprootedness
Unequal opportunity	Drop in self-esteem	Marginalization
Suffering	Loss of control	Criminality
		Violence
		Suicide

Exclusion is a trauma that is expressed over the short and long terms
in accordance with the child's character.

NEW ROLES FOR PEDIATRICIANS

There is very little in the scientific literature about the role of
physicians, whether preventive or curative, in community activities, and less still regarding psychosocial or economic factors that influence children's health. In this domain, the
physician has traditionally intervened as soon as someone
gets "hurt," whether through an injury caused by an accident
or an incident of intoxication, or through delayed growth resulting from family problems or a developmental problem of
psychosocial origin. There is little incentive for a physician to

become more involved in new roles from the financial stand-point, and medical training does not prepare doctors to un-dertake this type of intervention. The best interests of the child and the new needs children have today require a change in practice to deal with the causes and determinants of health problems. Experience has demonstrated the effec-tive role pediatricians can play in fostering this openness among medical practitioners.

For example, the American Academy of Pediatrics' Com-mon Access to Child Health (CATCH) program, which is designed to improve health care for children, enlisted pedia-tricians along with other members of the community to solve children's health problems through the use of local re-sources. A study of pediatricians in Colorado who partici-pated in the program[13] found that a large proportion had volunteered for activities and given their time to clinics for underprivileged children or recreational programs. The au-thor reported a high rate of satisfaction among pediatricians who participated, noting that they had a real interest in in-vesting their time along with other members of the commu-nity to meet the needs of children.

There is great potential for pediatricians in joining a collec-tive effort to provide care to children. It·only remains for each doctor to take the initiative and find ways to facilitate this movement towards children's local environments, whether as a way of protecting children, preventing health problems, or treating chronic illnesses. The future and credibility of pediat-rics are at stake, and this responsibility rests on the entire soci-ety. If all sectors of society participate in helping children and communities in every way, the service will become much more appropriate and more effective. Pediatricians certainly play a key role in the evolution of care for children.

Supporting the Family

A great variety of family support programs are found in com-munities in response to growing problems that sometimes leave families unable to fulfill their parental obligations. The most effective programs are those that tend to reinforce the family's abilities and take steps to foster the child's development through measures that affect various facets of their everyday life. The social pediatrician has a responsibility to interact with this type of valuable resource in the community. In a 1995 article,[14] the Committee on Early Childhood of the American Academy of Pediatrics made the following recommendations:

1 Pediatricians should be sensitive to all the problems families are facing and learn to recognize situations that interfere with effective parenting practices;
2 Pediatricians should be able to give families a warm welcome by forming special confidential links on an ongoing basis to promote an open discussion of needs, expectations, and ways of overseeing the child's development, as well as supporting parenting abilities;
3 The type of support the pediatrician gives parents should be based on a relationship of collaboration and shared decision-making so that the parents feel more competent or actually become more competent (i.e., a real partnership);
4 The pediatrician should refer to community-based groups and programs to help the parents to upgrade their knowledge and abilities so they can take charge of their children (i.e., empowerment). In some cases, the pediatrician may even develop such programs;
5 The pediatrician's participation in community-based family support programs makes it possible to offer expert advice on the health and safety of children in terms of organizing services and technical information parents need. This gives the pediatrician an opportunity to learn how to make a greater contribution to joint efforts of children, families and communities – a true community pediatrics;
6 The pediatrician should get involved with communities in planning services better adapted to families and children who most need support.

The pediatrician's rapport with the family is derived from a redefinition of the caregiver-patient roles in which the hierarchy is eliminated and a two-way confidential relationship is established. This is the base of a partnership and complicity that shares the objective of working for children's health and well-being. The result fosters a greater sensitivity to the needs of children in their own milieu and a sharing of responsibilities and tasks that aim to do better for the child. Seen from this perspective, assistance and support programs are developed by a consensus of all the players, in addition to being more numerous and sustained.

Let's take the simple example of a pediatrician in contact with a family for a particular problem – a child who is having tantrums (crying jags) whenever he feels frustrated. If the doctor can obtain a consensus on what attitudes each member of the family should consistently take when the problem arises, a solution is near and the child is reassured. A child who gets clear signals, clearly delineated limits, and a consistent attitude from the parents, instead of ambiguous, intolerant, or contradictory messages, can develop harmoniously. As a figure of great credibility, the pediatrician can and should have an influence on the family, along with the community and the family's beliefs.

Detecting Problems

The pediatrician's place within the family, especially in a support role recognized by the parents, makes the doctor a privileged partner in detecting the first signs of problems a child may be having with development, behaviour, or emotions. Knowing how important nonphysical problems can be, pediatricians can anticipate their potential long-term consequences if the problems pass unnoticed or unaddressed. So the pediatrician takes action, remaining in frequent contact with the parents, asking the right questions about the child's development and behaviour, and carefully observing the parent-child relationship. The pediatrician must be able to develop effective strategies for identifying and understanding the causes and symptoms of a child's psychosocial problems. Such strategies include the use of validated screening questionnaires, techniques for interviewing the parents and children, direct observation of the parent-child relationship in the office or in the family environment (at school, at home, at the recreation centre or daycare), and analyzing the parents' behaviour.

Several questionnaires primarily used for research can be adapted for use as clinical guides to detect children's behavioural and emotional problems. The Child Behavior Checklist, the Pediatric Symptoms Checklist, and the Conners can also be used by clinicians to complete the child's overall assessment, along with the Denver Developmental Screening Test (DDST), used in screening for developmental problems, and the Diagnostic and Statistical Manual of Mental Disorders Primary Care (DSM-PC), for psychosocial problems.

Studies have shown,[15] for example, that only thirty percent of pediatricians use a formal test such as the DDST to evaluate children's development. However, relying only on subjective clinical judgments formed in the office is acknowledged to be an imprecise method that can lead to inappropriate labelling of children and even false prognoses.

There is no such thing as a perfect test, and all tests should be used in conjunction with seasoned clinical and social judgment.[16] Coupled with the use of tools such as questionnaires, observation of parental behaviour and the parent-child relationship will likely not only detect problems but also move the parent-pediatrician partnership to a new level in caring for the child. While direct observation may take place in a neutral setting such as the doctor's office or the hospital, there are serious limitations to such sites given the inherent constraints of time allotments, for example, or the obvious patient-professional hierarchy. The professional may want to "show off" his or her competence; the patient may also want to put on a good show, which would naturally falsify the results. It is therefore a good idea in many cases to extend the observation to a natural setting, playing a direct role by visiting the home, school, or daycare, or teaming up with community partners who are privy to information through their daily contact with the child or family.

This direct presence is helpful in validating formal tools by comparing them with the child's everyday circumstances in order to get a full, objective profile of the child's state of health and development – the dynamic image of the child in his or her environment. This method is much more compatible with the global approach, in which the child is at the centre of a multifaceted environment with all the facets in continuous interaction.

Whether the purpose is to detect problems, evaluate the situation, or plan an intervention for a child who has a communication or developmental problem or a chronic condition, it is crucial to go beyond a simple static observation, a one-way mirror study in an office or hospital, or an assessment of the child's life at a given time. You need to see the child in action in real time and in his or her own space from day to day. The pediatrician in the community can serve as a relay point for such dynamic observations, which are beneficial to the child.

In some cases, several hours may be spent with a multidisciplinary team in a specialized hospital setting to diagnose a severe communication problem, such as autism. Doing this in isolation would entail the risk of failing to obtain essential dynamic information from the family and the environment, precipitating a serious diagnosis that could be compromising for the child based on momentary "appearances," and suddenly demobilizing the family as a partner because everything is happening too fast and they are finding it hard to follow. If the child is also from a different cultural community or has suffered major trauma (e.g., war, maltreatment, violence), or if the family is hiding dark secrets, conducting an assessment in isolation is even more risky and could lead to an incomplete diagnosis – and, worst of all, the demobilization of the family. The full extent of suffering associated with the symptoms may not be recognized; it may not even come to light. How can anyone act effectively under such conditions?

We often see in the clinic children who have been diagnosed as "hyperactive" and put on a serious drug regimen, when the symptom is only the manifestation of a malaise that may never be identified. All too often, behavioural problems in children or teens lead to exclusion or punishment when they are really a cry for help – but no one is listening and giving the child the treatment he or she needs. *The pediatrician's role is to make sure that all children can be understood, that their symptoms are properly decoded, and that justice and equity prevail in the services they receive.*

Tackling Psychosocial Problems

Since not all pediatricians have an interest in psychosocial problems, various initiatives have been taken to try to arouse their interest. In a study on pediatricians' involvement in psychosocial problems, McCue Horwitz et al.[17] reported an identification rate on the order of 27.3 percent for children between the ages of four and eight. The most commonly detected problems were family problems, such as divorce or conflict between the parents; behavioural problems, such as bed wetting and crying jags; learning problems; and attention disorders. On the other hand, the authors noted that parent-child relationship problems, conduct disorders, and peer relationship problems were underidentified. Aggressiveness and delinquent behaviour in boys are also more frequently recognized than anxiety and depression in girls. According to the study, pediatricians provided services either directly or by recommendation to more than half of the children in whom they detected a problem of this nature. The problems reported were moderate or major, while those described as slight were ignored or handled by the pediatrician.

The study had its limitations, as it focused on a restricted number of pediatricians in a particular place, so there is no point in generalizing these data to cover the whole profession. However, experience would seem to bear out the statistics. We can clearly do better at handling children's psychosocial problems, from identifying the problem to taking charge, if we hope to have a positive impact on the child's life trajectory.

The authors suggest that the type of visit, the time allotted, and the depth of the problem, as well as the pediatrician's knowledge of the child and family in terms of continuity, should influence the quality of screening for psychosocial problems and how they are handled. I would add that, given the complexity of these problems and the many causal factors, pediatricians should also develop deep tentaclelike roots in the child's milieu and form partnerships with the community and professionals from other disciplines and sectors. This global network-based approach is the only way to ensure the quality and effectiveness of professional care when it comes to complex problems in children. In this spirit, a friend of the child in question may contribute relevant information on the quality and problems of the child's peer relationships. A neighbour or social worker may provide an explanation of an opposition problem due to difficult parent-child relationships. The school or community groups can promote the establishment of measures that can bring a child out of suicidal isolation or help him or her to return to school. Nothing must be overlooked in assessing a child – especially not the child's connections with his or her own networks.

In this field, no one works alone. Interacting with the milieu and activating support networks are essential to the child's well-being. This is how the pediatrician becomes more sensitive to psychosocial problems and helps to find lasting solutions for the child.

Preventing Violence

Violence and its implications for the child are now recognized as a real public health issue in which prevention has an important role to play.[18] Risk factors and trajectories of violence are clearly identified in the scientific literature, and this is where the pediatrician comes in. Violence frequently originates in childhood and is activated in adolescence. A continuum has also been shown to exist between behavioural problems in children and delinquency and violence at a later stage. This "continuity" in the trajectory of violence sends out a ray of hope that preventive action, if taken soon enough, can counter the trend. Armed with this knowledge, the pediatrician can intervene to promote the well-being of the children, working from a health-promotion perspective to attenuate risk factors and boost protective factors.

In cases of delinquency and violence, parental problems, poorly managed conduct disorders, social stress, school problems, and poverty[19] are among the major recognized risk factors. The family structure (single parent, separated, or divorced), socioeconomic difficulties, and the parent's personal problems have an indirect effect – acute at times – on parental abilities. But parental attitudes really have a direct influence on the child's equilibrium and how the child learns to handle social rules. These attitudes include lack of supervision, conflicts between the parents, rules that are ambiguous (i.e., not clearly stated) or exaggerated, inappropriate expectations, or excessive discipline, which serves as an incubator for violence and makes it more likely that the cycle of violence will continue. When these "parental factors" coexist with school problems, peer rejection, and a string of failures, it will not be long before the child seeks out traumas associated with delinquency to derive some meaning from all this. An unstable family base and exclusion by schoolmates or playmates of the same age, teachers, and the community will fuel low self-esteem, rejection of social norms, and attraction to antisocial and deviant behaviours that lead to violence or delinquency. Research has shown[20] that thirty-eight percent of children identified as aggressive in kindergarten were experiencing academic failure three years later – which clearly makes them excellent candidates for delinquency and violence.

The objective is to take action before problems develop, at a time when the child is certainly fragile but prevention still has a grip – instead of resorting to belated programs designed to reduce violence and crime, which are known to be only marginally effective, with a success rate of approximately ten percent. The pediatrician in the milieu is well placed to identify this type of problem very early on. Other studies have demonstrated the effectiveness of early intervention in improving parental attitudes, even during times of stress, and preventing aggressive behaviours in very young children – in fact, the younger the child, the more effective the intervention. Pediatricians need to promote the establishment of parent support programs in the community, with the goal of taking preventive action and having a positive impact on the trajectory of troubled children.

There are already some pilot programs, such as the program set up by Patterson et al.,[21] which teaches parents of children who display antisocial behaviour five basic skills for improving their relationship:

1 Show an interest in what the child is doing.
2 Supervise the child's behaviour.
3 Set clear rules and apply them consistently.
4 Set up a system of rewards and consequences based on behaviour.
5 Learn to negotiate disagreements so problems don't escalate.

Teaching parents these lessons is not a matter of spending five or ten minutes with them in an office. It requires direct contact with the parent, spread over many hours. Using the Patterson technique, Montreal researchers[22] conducted a study involving parents and teachers of children in a high-risk kindergarten class showing disruptive behaviour. The intervention proved to be effective in: 1) reducing pushy behaviour at the age of nine; 2) encouraging eleven-year-olds to admit to being involved in a fight; and 3) committing teachers to report (rather than ignore) twelve-year-olds having a fight. In addition, from the age of twelve, these boys were less likely to be involved in breaking and entering and theft, and less prone to overconsumption than the control group.

The skills listed by Patterson (see above) can also be applied to improve adult-child relationships in schools and other settings where children learn to live happily as functional members of society. The pediatrician's role involves, at the very least, promoting adults' interest in these children, particularly in what they are doing, who they are, and what they will become. Children in whom someone shows an interest do not feel rejected and are able to develop in a harmonious way.

The pediatrician can also help find overall support for families with problems and be involved in promoting good habits and parenting abilities.[23] Social isolation and social stress are major risk factors that lead to violence and child neglect. It is imperative to take preventive action on these factors to understand their causes and strengthen the family. A number of programs established in the community provide support for families: information programs, such as parent support programs; emotional support programs, such as integrated home programs; instrumental programs that provide food support or adequate housing; and respite programs (daycare and respite centres). To date, the best results have been achieved through integrated programs based on meeting various types of needs at the same time by enlisting significant figures in the child's environment.

The pediatrician can identify families that need social support very early on and convince them to make use of existing support services, referring them to community groups that provide appropriate support in a respectful way. It is important for the pediatrician to know what preventive programs are in place in the community, or at least make sure that such programs are available in the milieu. He or she should also make sure that there is continuity with families in terms of motivation and oversee the progress of the children, above all ensuring that these children have access to protective measures against violence, such as those identified by Werner and Smith in a twenty-year observation study of children living in a poor and disadvantaged neighbourhood.[24] The authors found the following traits, which constitute factors that prevent the emergence of violence:

- the availability in the family of a significant adult besides the mother (father, grandparent, or older child);
- how much attention the child receives from the significant person in early childhood;
- the structure and rules in the milieu during adolescence;
- the cohesion of the family;
- the presence of an informal network of relatives and friends during adolescence.

The determinants of violence have a cumulative effect, especially in early childhood and throughout the perinatal period.[25] Ways of countering violence are well known: everything must be put in place so that children are loved, guided, and appreciated, in suitable settings and right from the first years of life, if we really want to act in the best interests of the child.

A Noble and Political Role

Beyond the traditional role of diagnosing and treating illness, the social pediatrician is in a position to carve out a broader role in meeting children's needs by taking up their cause. This means becoming more involved in children's lives by keeping tabs on the factors that determine their state of health and making sure that someone is keeping an eye on them. The pediatrician should focus on children's emotional, psychological, cultural, and social problems, as well as their physical problems, since everything is related and modulated in the family and the milieu.[26] The medical approach absolutely must be changed to become more sensitive to risk factors that are present in the child's circle. The pediatrician's mission must be redefined to include the ability to take preventive action to reinforce various protective factors that boost the child's well-being and intervene in a more appropriate way that is in harmony with the family and the milieux. The doctor should become a catalyst for joint action with communities to support children's health and even become the prime promoter of the best interests of the child with parents, families, communities, and the political system.

With parents and other adults, the pediatrician can provide a fix on how the child is developing – what is equitable and good for the child. The doctor can also guide a parent with problems to an appropriate resource or adapted therapy program to protect the child from consequences that could impede his or her development.

With families, the pediatrician can serve as an intermediary, guide, or reference person, encouraging the mother, father, or other member of the extended family to participate. In a crisis, the doctor can point the way to family therapy or even find role models for the child. The level of involvement can be high but should always take place in an atmosphere of respect and partnership for the well-being of the child.

With communities, the pediatrician is in a position to oversee the establishment of quality resources designed to support children and families, motivating local players to develop mutual support networks, and sometimes even personally organizing effective care through complete adapted services in the child's own milieu.

Overall, social pediatricians will now be recognized by governments and society as advocates for children's health, taking clear positions to influence policies, legislation, and programs that affect children's health and their best interests.

PART TWO

The Practice of Social Pediatrics

ACTS OF HEALING

Pediatricians practise pediatrics. Social pediatricians stick their noses into anything and everything that can help children, especially children in distress. This may lead to accusations of not "minding your own business," being too "pro-family," or "failing to follow procedures." I have been the target of every one of those accusations myself. But should we abstain from intervening if the measures required to help a needy child involve something special, something that is not "usual"? Especially when we know what a difference it can make to the child throughout his or her life?

The stories in this section of the book are based on my own experience in the practice of social pediatrics. Recently, as a way of explaining what I do, I have tried to take notes – for example, on a touching interview with one child or the story of another child who completely bowled me over. I have tried to describe what happened in each case so that readers can understand the scope of our work and the full impact that we – parents and professionals – can have on the child we are hoping to help – as long as we know how to listen to the child, understand, and then take action.

I have tried to use these real-life stories to illustrate what we must to do to help children who are suffering from various forms of trauma and rejection and who are living in appalling conditions. Most of these children are right in our midst, but as long as we fail to reach out to them, we have no idea what they are going through. And we simply don't see how essential our help can be.

I have no illusions about remaking society, but I hope that this book – and especially the children's own stories – can help us draw upon the more humanistic elements to realize that children, if we just give them the chance, have the capacity to restore their own equilibrium quite quickly. I do not pretend to be a problem-solving missionary or magician. Fleeting illusions are not my stock-in-trade. All the same, this approach does contain a healthy dose of spirituality – or at least, something that elevates human nature, makes people open and available, and spurs them on to achieve great things. Sometimes it is just such partners, coming from unexpected quarters, who devise solutions that turn out to have nearly magical effects.

I hope the children's stories will serve as a concrete illustration of the EEDA method discussed in Part One:

- ESTABLISHING a special relationship;
- EXCHANGING information;
- DECODING knowledge and experience; and
- ACTION based on a consensus between family members and professionals.

While the outcome of these cases is filtered through the lens of social pediatrics, it is certainly not the sole province of pediatricians. The actions that really make a difference are those that are taken in the child's world and by the child's family and friends – everyone who has an influence on the child, as a role model, parent, disciplinary figure, teacher, coach, or guide. A physician with deep roots in the community who is open to this type of approach can play the dual role of conductor and moderator, weaving together bits of information from various sources and pointing in the right direction so that appropriate action can be taken.

The conductor of an orchestra must be familiar with each piece of music and know where each instrument comes in – as well as understanding the deeper meaning of the composition. Similarly, professionals need to understand what the child *means* in his or her natural milieu – in other words, where the child belongs in the centre of a universe that provides the support the child needs to survive and grow up. Most of all, the professional-*cum*-conductor needs to detect the intimate mechanisms that promote the child's harmonious development. This is essentially a two-step process. The first step involves immersion in the dynamic processes of the child and the family to find the deeper causes of the problem, based on the symptoms. The second step involves finding mechanisms that will help the child to become healthy again and find new meaning in life. Of course, the process may also involve a wide range of mechanisms and tools, such as specific recreational activities, therapy, and even medication if necessary.

What really matters is making sure that all these steps lead concurrently to a single goal: to find and fan the flame of that little light that shines in every child's eyes – however faint or deeply concealed it may sometimes be – for that ever-burning flame is what truly gives us hope.

The first three chapters of this segment of the book deal with the search for feelings, identity, and meaningful connections. Please bear in mind that it is crucial to decode the deeper meaning of the signs and symptoms children show, which generally relate to "big" feelings and fundamental needs. This dynamic approach is what social pediatrics is all about.

CHAPTER FIVE

The Search for Feelings

MARK — DIAGNOSIS: BROKEN HEART

I was quite surprised the first time I met Mark, a lively, voluble, intelligent nine-year-old. Clearly concerned about his image, he was well dressed and groomed, with clean, well-cut hair. Quite a contrast to his mother, a frail, nervous young woman with rings on every finger, not to mention in her ears and through her nose. However, I could see that their relationship was extremely close. Why had they come to see me? Mark didn't look sick at all. In fact, he was a breath of fresh air.

It took a while for the problem to surface. After chatting pleasantly for a few minutes about nothing in particular (as usual at this stage), Mark finally told me what the matter was. He was heartsick, missing his dear friend Isabelle. She'd gone away six months before, but he just couldn't seem to get over it. Once the problem was out in the open, he had no trouble talking. He couldn't stop thinking about her, day and night, though he'd had no word of her for six months. One day in the schoolyard she told him that her family was moving to another part of town. For Mark, it was a catastrophe. He hadn't seen her since, but she was in his thoughts all day long and in his dreams every night. She was his best friend, he said, the one who understood him best and really listened to him. Mark's life had nearly ground to a halt. At school, his marks, always excellent, had plummeted; it took him forever to get to sleep, and he had lost interest in everything he used to enjoy. But when he spoke of Isabelle his face lit up, his eyes shone, and he was full of life.

Mark was in mourning, and he could see no end to it. Isabelle must be a wonderful girl to inspire such deep feelings in such a young boy, I thought. While some might dismiss his pain, I knew that it was very serious. The importance of this type of sadness, which can lead to all sorts of problems even at such a tender age, should never be minimized.

Was he depressed or suicidal? What could we do to get this boy back on track? This was a crucial period in his development, when his health and well-being could be at risk. But why come to see a doctor who was supposed to treat physical problems? Mark and his mother were clearly expecting me to come up with some solution. Perhaps more specialized treatment was needed. Was I the right person to take care of this child? What was I getting into here? I realized that the decision to come to me with the problem had not been taken lightly, as the two of them had discussed it at length before confiding in me. The decision to consult me in particular was also premeditated – a relative had urged them to talk it over with me. So what could I do but try my best to help? At least I could take the first steps. If necessary, I could refer them to someone else later on, but for now I could not betray their confidence and lose momentum by failing to take immediate action.

I listened to Mark's story, heard his pain, and welcomed his confidence. I suggested that he write a letter to Isabelle telling her how much distress she had inadvertently caused him. I said that perhaps she was just as unhappy without him in her new neighbourhood, at school, and at home. Although he didn't know where she lived or went to school, we would try to find her, and when the letter reached her she would realize how much he cared. Now that I had won his trust, Mark began to tell me complicated stories about the moon and the stars, complete with pictures. It didn't mean much to me at the time, although he was trying to make me understand. Reassured, he left totally transformed, and we agreed to meet again soon.

When he returned a few weeks later, Mark was radiant, full of life and a new sense of direction. He had come to tell me that everything was fine, he had written the letter, and life was good again. That was all he said. What had really happened? Why had I been given the privilege of sharing the immeasurable pain of love with a boy of nine? What had I done to help? What button had I pushed to help him get back on track? It would remain a mystery.

The "human" approach sometimes guards such secrets, and we should not try to probe them. The lack of scientific explanation is a good thing in this case. Why attempt to dissect something that is fundamentally very simple when the best solution is listening with compassion? For Mark, the first stage – establishing a relationship – meant confiding in me and sharing powerful emotions. That was what he was hoping for when he decided to share his great secret with me – a doctor and a total stranger. I did not deny or minimize his pain but welcomed and shared it. He could tell that my interest was sincere, although I clearly didn't understand it all, especially when he tried to explain it in another dimension – a dimension of stars and moons and dreams. This rapprochement, this attempt to understand, meant that we could work together in a concerted way to come up with some simple solutions that would dissipate his pain and set the healing process in motion. It hadn't taken Mark long to find an accomplice and come back to earth, to find meaning in this emotion that was too big for him and go back to being a boy of nine who was growing up. As for me, I had met a little prince in love, who had won my heart.

MAX – HOLDING BACK THE TEARS

Eight-year-old Max never cried. He told me so right off the bat in a clear, firm voice. His first visit seemed rather surrealistic.

Max came in with his mother, a woman in her early twenties. His school had sent him to see me for concentration problems.

Behind his self-confident façade Max seemed sad, pale, and puffy-eyed. He was visibly agitated. His mother shyly told me her story. She was working as a call girl for an escort service. She had a drug abuse problem and was living on her own with Max at the moment. She wasn't really sure who the father was. She'd had a rough life herself, including sexual violence, incest, foster homes, many moves, and various forms of rejection. She described her family background as "very difficult," with major losses that dated back for several generations. The child had witnessed sordid scenes, from violence to attempted murder of family members. This is the type of severe trauma children of war experience – only this time, it was happening in Montreal.

Max, an intelligent interesting kid, never cried. Children – or big kids, at least – don't cry, he said. Everyone knew that. His mother reported that sometimes he did very well at school, but there were other times when things were harder for him, he wouldn't listen to anyone or anything, was not open to learning, and seemed to be "not quite there." With his mother, he could be quite charming, attentive, and obliging, but sometimes living together was hell for both of them.

Max's mother had been trying to rebuild her life for some time. She had signed up for courses, joined support groups, and was hoping to find a more regular job soon. However, Max had recently become more difficult and disorganized. He was always worrying about his mother. He was upset about not seeing her at lunchtime – he stayed at school for lunch now – and panicked if she was late by even a few minutes. We've seen this before many times, of course: when the mother progresses, the baby regresses. He wasn't doing well in class, becoming very demanding and aggressive. The slightest frustration sent him into a tailspin. As his mother grew through these new experiences, Max stagnated, making no progress, even regressing. That was the most disturbing part.

No, he never shed a tear – but while we were talking, his eyes frequently filled up. His eyes were puffy from the effort not to cry; he was obviously very sad and in deep distress. On his slender shoulders he bore sorrows that dated back several generations. Thanks to his solid, loving relationship with his mother, he had managed to survive, function normally, and cope with life. But now his cup was full and his eyes were on the verge of spilling over. His mother was changing, she wasn't always there, and she was not in such great need of his protection. Their roles were changing, and Max had to face up to the reality of his own life. Most of all, he needed to learn to cry. My role had suddenly become clear – I was there to give him "permission" to cry. And those tears would do him so much good.

My true role as an accomplice and witness to great secrets was emerging. I was now an actor in the trajectory of a child in distress. Knowing the family had confidence in me and had given me this "job," I felt I was entitled to take action. Would it be appropriate to hand Max over to someone he didn't know at this point? Would he ever confide in me again if I were to do so? All right – my path was clear.

Of course Max needed to let himself cry, but the main thing he had to do was accept his many losses and grieve for them. His major "bereavement" – the sorrow that was blocking his development – was the way his mother was changing. For him, this was the equivalent of a fresh loss. He needed to discharge his sorrow by changing the way he dealt with things: he needed to become the agent of his own development rather than his mother's protector. He needed to form an affiliation, or rather reaffiliate in a consistent and secure way, with the person who was nearest and dearest to him – his own mother. He needed to make the effort to resume his childhood trajectory at the appropriate developmental stage for his age. His mother had work to do as well. Despite her current fears and problems, she needed to pursue her own path without feeling guilty and realize that was the best way to provide positive support for her child and make their

attachment more secure. What a contract between a child
who had already suffered too many emotional wounds and a
young mother few would give much of a chance!

The professional here, knowing the family secrets, realiz-
ing what was at stake and what events can place a child at
risk, had a clear role to play: setting in motion various mechanisms to support the child and his mother, with respect and
confidence, and help them improve their lives. There was no
question here of taking the easy way out and just writing a
prescription, a therapy that is overused today for this type of
problem. When a child shows confidence, we must *reinforce
that confidence*, provide intensive accompaniment, promote
significant attachments, and get the child back on the trajectory to harmonious development. Here was the action plan:

1 *Reinforce confidence*: Stay in close contact with the child, not
   divulging his secrets, but using those secrets to take action
   on his behalf. This could take the form of brief regular
   meetings in various settings, such as the clinic, school, or
   home, where exchanges could take place through games,
   drawings, and words. I saw Max again several times at home.
   He showed me his room and his things – his favourite toys
   and books. I saw him at community lunches organized by
   the Pop-mobile (a project in Montreal that provides free
   lunches and a place to go for children in the underprivileged neighbourhood of Hochelaga-Maisonneuve). I also
   saw him again several times at the clinic. As his confidence
   grew, he found many new courses of effective action rooted
   in his daily life.
2 *Provide intensive accompaniment:* Be with the child in his own
   community with the people in his regular circle. In this
   case, school was the best place, since that was where Max's
   problems had first been noticed. Once we understand the
   child's suffering, we can develop many types of support
   that will help the child refocus – through strict attitudes
   and models, but most of all through compassion. Having
   lunch with the street workers from the Pop-mobile pro-

vided a further opportunity to mobilize significant figures to act on the child's behalf and show their support by making small yet important gestures. It was also very important to be there to accompany the tormented dynamic of the mother-son relationship in this difficult adjustment period by supporting the mother personally and reassuring her that what she was doing would be of benefit to her child. This could take the form of providing emotional and psychological assistance or temporary help in the form of food, furniture, or money to reduce her stress, or it could mean finding respite care to let her "catch her breath" and get a few hours to herself.

3 *Allow significant attachments:* In a way, this means promoting the rapprochement of adults around the child so that they develop a secure attachment model (as we saw in the section on attachment, this is very important). This sends a clear signal that an adult who is close to the child should if possible provide a reassuring emotional connection that will serve as a beacon, guide, and reference point for a fixed period, giving him time to rebuild his regulatory mechanisms and get his trajectory back on course. For a child like Max, this means being able to feel safe with an adult for the first time in his life. This is also the best way for him to learn how to rebuild a solid attachment with his mother and develop models that could serve as a reference point for the future to protect him from new problems and sorrows, getting him back on his developmental track.

For Max's mother, who lived in difficult conditions and had never known attachment or security herself, these steps would strengthen her aspirations for a better life, which would probably be more difficult for her to achieve on her own. The significant adult-child-parent alliance that was created would continue long enough to allow the parent-child relationship to refocus.

We see this type of case in the clinic quite often, but unfortunately not many professionals are willing to "get on board."

Many children feel insecure about their community and their family. Insecurity produces all sorts of upheavals in terms of the child's development, behaviour, or adaptation. The traditional intervention process has an unfortunate tendency to react to such symptoms in a punitive manner, through expulsion or other forms of withdrawal and consequences that only serve to reinforce the sense of insecurity. What we need to do is set in motion interventions that will provide a sense of security. This does necessarily not rule out certain unpleasant consequences, but it is part of a global process that allows the child to refocus and the parent to reappropriate his or her role as a secure guide. This can only be done through a method that involves establishing a special relationship, exchanging, decoding, and taking action in partnership with the child's circle: our EEDA approach.

Bit by bit, Max learned how to cope with his situation, thanks to several supportive adults who came to a consensus for joint action – and most of all, made themselves available to Max. Whenever his mother was having a hard time, someone (a person or a group) from the circle would take over – take him to sports or another recreational activity, invite him to stay for a few days, or give the mother a chance to "vent." During one especially difficult time for Max and his mother, a volunteer took him home with her for a whole week so he could see how a supervised family setting really works. Max's mother sometimes consulted the family for reassurance and tips on things to do with her son.

The school pitched in, too, aware of the possible risk for the child if sustained action was not taken promptly. When Max was going through a rough time and lashing out to provoke rejection, just the opposite would happen. He would be taken to the office and face certain consequences, but someone was always with him, working through his problem and helping him to understand. The active participation of the school in such a process of helping is essential. This requires establishing a relationship between professionals and, most of all, a common goal of doing whatever it takes to help the child. And it works.

A year or so later, Max was a changed child, always the first to help, caring about others and able to talk. I suspected that he was even able to cry when needed – but that was private territory. His mother had gone back to school to study hair-dressing, with plans to open her own salon one day.

Children are human beings in mutation. They need guides, reference points, and role models – and most of all, they have a great need to talk about their troubles, and cry if they want to.

DANIEL – FINDING THE STRENGTH TO SAY GOODBYE TO HIS MOTHER

It took several meetings with Daniel before I realized why he was having so much trouble at school. Nine-year-old Daniel was very sweet, pleasant, and endearing, but according to the adults in his life, he was in a constant state of motion – turning, twirling, bustling about. It was dizzying to watch, but he was not hyperactive. Actually, he seemed worried and preoccupied, rather distant. My first impression was that he was miles away.

Daniel lived with his grandparents, his grandmother serving as a substitute for his absent mother. Daniel adored and respected her and seemed extremely attached to her. She appeared to be rather overwhelmed and distraught but also showed great tenderness towards the child. Right from our very first meeting, it was obvious that even the slightest mention of his real mother aroused strong feelings of great sadness for both the child and his grandmother. Daniel would become even more agitated and evasive, trying to get up and leave. His grandmother seemed confused and at a loss for words, a sign of great distress.

After a while, I learned that the absent mother had enormous problems. She had no fixed address and wandered the streets, a victim of drug abuse and HIV. Her rare contacts with her family were nearly always made in the most impersonal way, by telephone. I also learned that Daniel was always worrying about his mother, afraid that something might happen to her and that he would never see her again, that she might disappear forever or be unable to cope with her suffering. But the main thing I learned was that Daniel's despair was eating away at him. His strong sense of loyalty to his mother, despite her absence, was stalling his development and blocking his attachment to his grandparents, who were very kind to him. I found out that twice he had seen his mother on the street by accident – and what was really awful was that when they saw each other and hope dawned in both their eyes, she ran away. Daniel was inconsolable. For several years he had lived in this ambiguous situation, which would be intolerable for anyone, but especially for a young child.

What I have found most striking over the course of my career working with children in distress is the strong emotional connection between parent and child, which is usually composed of unforgettable times and shared joys but is sometimes attenuated by ambiguities that are intolerable for both parent and child. Many sorrows and health problems arise from what is *not said* between parent and child – the evasions and prevarications. Professionals need to be attentive to this when they are trying to find the real reasons why a child or teen is having such a hard time. Sometimes it's an absent or inconsistent father, who makes all sorts of promises but never keeps them. More often, a visceral fear born of insecurity makes the child fear that he will lose his mother, that she will fall ill or die, just not come home from work one day, or be kidnapped. And that fear invariably arises from a lack of clarity and communication, on the pretext of protecting the child from a truth considered too much for the child to bear. What really is too much for the child to bear and does a great deal of harm, however, is not the truth but *hiding the truth*.

For Daniel, it was clearly time to take action, so we made a pact – the grandmother, Daniel, and I. We agreed to try to arrange a meeting between the three of us and the mother, to talk or at least, I thought, share some feelings or perhaps draw some connections between what everyone was going through. The grandmother's job was to make it clear to her daughter at the first opportunity that she had to agree to talk about her son and eventually meet face to face and do some explaining. For the grandmother and Daniel, the agreement brought fresh hope, though both were still struggling with deep sadness. My role was becoming clearer: I would be a sort of mediator-*cum*-accomplice for them, trying to crystallize or exorcise their sorrows. Since the mother was on the streets and in great distress, we would all need to be patient and wait until she showed up again. And we would need to do some serious listening as we tried to find the right arguments that would convince her to meet our expectations. That was the most delicate and risky part of the whole story.

Our pact or agreement – our exercise in complicity – was already effecting a change in Daniel, based on hope, of course, but also re-establishing a more balanced developmental state. He was behaving differently at school. While we were waiting, his behaviour seemed to stabilize and his marks improved. He was also able to resume the recreational activities he had lost interest in and started hanging out with his friends again.

Several attempts proved to be fruitless, which was discouraging. Daniel had occasional relapses in behaviour and more trouble at school. I was still confident, stubbornly believing that it would be worthwhile and that the mother-daughter-son reunion was the only way to thwart the stifling feelings everyone was experiencing, which were disturbing the child so profoundly. I was a little worried about how we would proceed if the famous meeting finally occurred, especially how it would end, when everyone would of course be shattered by strong emotions. However, I was so convinced of the symbolic and beneficial importance of the event that I continued to support the child and the grandmother, hoping for a magical sort of spontaneous healing that would be difficult to reconcile with any scientific method.

In the practice of social pediatrics, sometimes events outstrip us, but as observers, we can regard the emotions in

question with some objectivity. On that basis, we can keep
hope alive and under the right conditions, provide *assurance*
that positive change will come about.

In this case, the most rational hypothesis involved shedding some light on the great ambiguity that surrounded the
roles of the major players in this drama and the identity
problems Daniel was experiencing. The only way he had
been able to express his suffering was by acting out to attract
attention. The proposed solution was simple, perhaps sim-
plistic: give all the players a chance to clarify a complex situation; invite the itinerant mother to give her son permission
to accept the grandmother as a substitute; get her to tell her
mother how happy she was to hand over that role; and finally, ask her to reassure Daniel that her love for him was unconditional, despite her current circumstances.

Then one day when we'd almost lost hope, the time came
– a memorable moment of pure joy. I came back from lunch
to find Daniel pacing anxiously in the waiting-room with his
grandmother. The first thing he asked me was whether I had
"seen her." I didn't understand what he meant until he repeated it twice. So the time had come. That morning, she
had phoned to see what was new and, against all expectations, agreed to come to a long-awaited meeting. She was already a few minutes late, but Daniel was sure that this time
she really would come. While we were waiting, he told me
that he'd seen her at the corner a few days before, but she
was probably feeling too emotional or hopeless, so she ran
away. He confessed that he had felt a great emptiness, but today he was sure she would come.

The joy was intense for everyone. We had been waiting
around the table for an hour when she appeared at the door,
frail, so thin you could almost see through her, excited,
graceful in a dress that was obviously second-hand but suited
her well. Everything was said in just a few words, interspersed
with great silences and a continuous flow of tears. It was an
unforgettable meeting for an emotional mother, her proud
son, and his grandmother, who was feeling great relief – the

kind of reunion you sometimes see after a separation of 20
or 40 years. The mother found happiness that day that she
had not believed possible. Daniel obviously took great pride
in his dazzling mother. He wanted to share her with everyone who hadn't seen her for months or years and had simply
lost hope of ever seeing her again. He wanted to take her to
visit the whole family circle, go to a restaurant, and enjoy the
rest of the fine Indian summer weather with her.

I made a few suggestions to the mother who was in a
trance, still trying to decide whether to leave or stay. I suggested that she give her son the pleasure of spending a few
minutes together at a café, face to face. They left, or rather
flew off, to mend their bridges, and I remained with a muted
image of a woman in agony, deeply hurt yet overjoyed, and a
child who was sad but renewed in his love for his mother.

We met again a few days later at the house. A family council
was held around the kitchen table. Now that his mother had
given permission, the main order of business was Daniel's
"adoption." She had vanished again after that happy flying
visit, but her work was done. Surrounding Daniel were his
grandparents, cousins, an aunt, a brother-in-law, and his sister,
who was not much older than Daniel but who already had a
baby of her own. Everyone around the table, in their own sub-
tle way, laid claim to the child, each stating their role. Daniel
could finally surrender to his real family, reassured, confident,
and liberated. It was another unforgettable moment, a time of
healing and integration that let Daniel refocus on his values
and attachments, so vital to his development.

A few months later, a meeting was held to discuss Daniel's
academic future. He was doing surprisingly well at school. All
the bigwigs from the school were united in praising his ex-
ceptional qualities as a human being as well as a student. The
people at that meeting, who had previously intervened to
help a little boy who was having problems, now congratu-
lated him in front of his grandmother, who was acknowledged as his new mother. She and Daniel were very proud to
hear their words of uncommon praise.

MARIE AND CHLOE —
A MATTER OF MODESTY

The behaviour and attitudes of these two girls seemed to suggest sexual abuse in the family. Marie and Chloe, two sisters who were very close, lived with their little brother and father in a rather isolated location. The father had been caring for the children on his own for nearly four years, following serious family problems associated with a situation that was critical for the children. They had been mistreated, physically and sexually, by people in the family circle some time earlier. Since then their father had assumed responsibility for providing a stable environment, but he was entirely cut off from the rest of the family and from outside influences.

While the father did have certain skills as an adult and a parent, he had some obvious intellectual limitations. He dressed like a tramp and had a mania for collecting all sorts of eccentric objects, which he kept in his cramped apartment. He also had trouble expressing himself coherently and was quite difficult to understand, especially in situations that were new to him. He had a facial tic and his body language revealed his shyness. Going strictly by appearances, few would judge him to be a competent parent.

In fact, however, the father was a clean, thrifty, resourceful, well-organized man. For example, he reduced the family electricity bill by unscrewing all the light bulbs but one at night. He could fix just about anything around the house, and his children were never lacking for the essentials of life. When he was with the children, he had a disturbing and unusual habit of throwing them penetrating glances, as if from amazement or envy. In a group, his bizarre attitudes clearly marked him as a deviant from normal social standards.

I believed that all these attitudes and behaviours revealed a certain malaise or discomfort. Was he actually content to observe others in an attempt to understand the customs and trends of society that he had never been able to learn? Perhaps he was trying to improve his own behaviour – who could say? While he had never been known to behave aggressively, he certainly made others feel uncomfortable to the point of leaving the room.

Marie, the eldest, was also very shy, with multiple developmental delays. In attitude and behaviour she resembled her father – head bowed, face sad, hesitant, and seemingly fearful. Excessive hair growth on her arms and legs caused her great distress since she was teased about it. That was the only subject that could really rouse her; her eyes would blaze with fury as she waited for someone to explain why it had to be that way.

Nine-year-old Chloe was different. When she was younger she had been rather reserved, but she had gradually turned into a determined, spirited, sarcastic, and happy young girl – at least that was how she looked. Recently, though, there had been another radical change: she dressed with great care, wore funky earrings, and was looking more and more like a responsible young adult who took pride in herself.

The family was certainly isolated, but several significant and supportive adults had helped the children over the past few years, both at school and in the community. The girls had no female role model at home, but they had managed to find role models in their everyday activities. Various people in the community had compensated for the children's isolation and lack of stimulation in such a fragile environment, attempting to provide the missing ingredients for their development. And the father, despite his self-imposed inaccessibility, had also earned a certain amount of respectful support from people who suspended judgment on his qualities as a parent and responsible adult.

Deceptive appearances to the contrary, there was a certain consensus in the milieu that the children deserved assistance and protection according to their needs. Everyone recognized that it was in the children's best interests for their father to take responsibility for them. Sometimes one community group would provide food or clothing while another got the children involved in sports or respite programs. When the father had something hard to do, there was always someone there beside him. At school, the children's behaviour and performance were monitored. Since all the professionals worked together from time to time, they would share bits of information, which helped everyone play their respective roles in maintaining the family's balance and ensuring the children's appropriate development. The father always accepted help gladly and was grateful for the consensus. In this case, the help they received meant that various interventions, such as placing the children, could be avoided. Placement would have been imposed from the outside with the same objective, the "best interests of the children." It all depends on our perspective and criteria for intervention.

But let's get back to our story. Recently, the neighbours had begun to worry about Marie and Chloe and their "sexual safety." The question was, was there something more, or something more intensive, that we (the responsible adults offering support) could do to support and protect the two girls in this family? Could we make sure that the girls were able to grow up in a harmonious way without being at risk? Could we somehow avoid exposing them to inappropriate or harmful situations that they might blame us for later on? We all know someone who was mistreated as a child and many years later complained that no one had taken the initiative or had the courage to help them when they really needed it. It was time to take action to avoid such a scenario and protect the children. The question was whether this was really indicated or how much doubt we were willing to tolerate. A serious question – and one we often hear in our clinical practice.

The neighbours' recent concerns were based on some peculiar circumstances. Some neighbours had complained that the curtains were drawn and the windows kept closed in the daytime, even in summer. Someone noticed that the children were never seen playing outside the house. Adults who had contact with the children were concerned and surprised at Marie's persistent shyness, the strange way they were dressed, and how they were easy targets for victimization by other children. Someone mentioned that the father, who was really rather strange-looking, kept on hanging around the school-yard. Others observed that Marie and Chloe seemed to be competing for their father: one was apparently entitled to presents (earrings and makeup) while the other was not; one would dress in an inappropriate manner for her age, while the other slept in the father's bedroom. Based on facts and observations, a possible scenario was born in the minds of well-intentioned people who wanted to "do the right thing."

So we held a "summit" of everyone who had contact with the father or the children to try to shed some light on the family situation, coordinate what we were doing with the family, and find more formal ways of protecting the children if necessary.

We concluded at the meeting that the father and children had access to continuous support from the community. They took part in recreational activities and someone was with them nearly every day. There were family visits, help from food banks, daycare, respite care, and more. We realized that all these programs, provided by all sorts of responsible people, did in fact provide stimulation, supervision, and appropriate role models for the children. We realized that the children had everything they needed, at home and in the community, to develop and blossom, or even confide in someone and get protection if they wanted – mainly thanks to the concrete attachment they had developed to some of those people. We were also sure that all these ongoing and intensive measures definitely contributed to the children's well-being and harmonious development, and that the habits that were deemed somewhat bizarre were nothing more than personal and "cultural" characteristics that were not of great importance. And we agreed that while the neighbours' opinions had been based on good faith, they were premature and without real foundation.

The consensus was that the family's support system was effective and provided sufficient protection. I believe that that consensus addressed the matter of reasonable doubt. If all the players share such a doubt, then we should acknowledge it. If they do not as a group believe that a real risk exists, forget it. Besides, with a network approach in which everyone plays his or her role properly, the risk of error is greatly reduced, and there is ongoing supervision in any case.

I was more convinced that the children were doing well when I saw them on their next visit to the clinic. I was impressed with both Marie and Chloe in terms of the questions they asked, and most of all, their modesty. They asked for explanations at each stage in the physical examination. They asked good questions and requested appropriate explanations. They were both extremely modest when it was time to examine their genitals. The entire visit was very respectful. I was particularly impressed by something Chloe said that showed how much she loved and understood her poor father and wanted to protect him. She told me, "When I grow up I'll move out, but I'll always come back to take care of my father."

Modesty, understanding, love, and respect are infallible indicators of a family's integrity and capacities – even if that family has problems and is "different," it is good enough. This story bears eloquent testimony to the confidence we need to have when working with families who are "different." And it also teaches us a lesson in respect and shows just how effective it can be to take joint action in the children's milieu. This is truly acting "in the best interests of the child."

PAUL — THE RIGHT TO BE ANGRY

Anger, like fear, is therefore articulated with the notion of an internal membrane that gives way under intense pressure. In fear ... it's the shell of the soul that opens accidentally and lets the core of the individual escape. In anger, it's the gall bladder that bursts, letting the bitter substance spread through the body, perhaps even making its way to the head to provoke a fit of rage.[1]

In my clinical practice, I have seen many children with every possible permutation of anger, their bodies trembling and voices shaking, obviously feeling utterly helpless. They lash out to provoke rejection, their suffering clearly so intense that it has become intolerable.

What struck me about Paul, who was eight years old, was just that permanent state of rage, ready to burst out at any moment and inundate those around him. To such an extent, in fact, that no one at school could tolerate him any more, and the only solution seemed to be to expel him to protect the other children – and the teachers. I was expressly asked to prescribe medication to control Paul's rage and stop him from endangering his own safety. At home, it was the same story. Her mother was at the end of her rope. Paul had declared war, he would not listen to anyone or anything – he had even managed to break his bed and smash the wall in his bedroom. Everyone called him a walking catastrophe.

Paul had been diagnosed with an attention disorder and behavioural problems. Questions had even been raised about his mental health. No one wanted to play with him, except for a few kids who would occasionally enlist him to start a fight or play some nasty tricks. But he was not violent or aggressive by nature. Uncontrollable rages would come on suddenly, transforming his personality. At school, his behaviour had become intolerable, and every conceivable solution had been tried: positive reinforcement, punishment, expulsion. A special tutor had been assigned to him without achieving any real results. A decision had just been made to suspend him on alternate days due to his "agitation, disobedience, and the threat he represents to others and to himself." The ultimatum was clear and direct: "no Ritalin, no school, except perhaps a special school for behavioural problems with a low ratio, for the next two weeks."

We see this type of diagnosis and "sentencing" regularly in pediatrics. In fact, this is often why we're asked to intervene. But where do we begin, really?

After my initial meeting with mother and child, I decided not to act too hastily – and especially not to label the child: he was already wearing too many labels, and labelling would be of absolutely no use in trying to help him. I didn't want to give too restrictive a treatment based on such scant information. My impressions and information were much too limited and biased to take action at this point. (Let's not forget the EEDA approach.)

One early indicator was quite important: the mother said that she was tired to the point of exhaustion. She had major problems herself, including drug dependency, and was barely able to look after herself at the moment. She confessed at our first meeting that she really needed help. But the key indicator that leapt out at me was the glaring absence of any sort of relationship between the mother and child. It wasn't just that there was coldness between them or that they ignored each others' presence: I could see that they were profoundly detached from each other. Both were clearly distressed, and it showed in their physical appearance and behaviour – the mother's emotional imbalance and the child's tantrums. But both bore their suffering alone, in total isolation. Based on this initial observation, it was clearly necessary to probe the deep-rooted reasons for the child's problems before attempting to offer any lasting solutions.

At this stage, my approach elicited only negative reaction from the school. They expected me to provide immediate solutions to the problem, not spout grand theories or prescribe lengthy therapy. They didn't want to see the child again unless he was on medication. They suggested sending him to a psychiatrist, subtly implying that I wasn't really competent to handle the case. (It was not the first time that had happened.) Such an attitude, which is quite common in some professionals or institutions – quickly referring the child outside the milieu – has definite limitations and is liable to harm the child, since it immediately eliminates any attempt to seek explanatory causes and codes that can explain children's problems. This can only lead to piecemeal measures that are unlikely to have lasting effects and can even cause certain conditions to deteriorate. If we are trying to take effective and coherent action, we must first place our trust in local resources, the parents, and community networks. More often than not, both explanations and solutions can be found locally.

I made another visit to Paul's home. He wasn't there, but it gave me the opportunity to see the sorry state of the poor mother, who had recently moved to a sparsely furnished apartment and was deeply distressed, fearful, and disorganized. She begged me to do something for Paul, frankly confessing that she was unable to take care of him and felt extremely guilty. She couldn't look him in the face and felt unable to take him in her arms, kiss him – love him as she had before. With too many emotional wounds of her own, she was asking for a truce, a time of respite to rebuild her strength and regain her balance. She asked me to explain all this to Paul without making him even more upset and find some way to help him. I had my work cut out for me.

The challenge was to find effective help in the network that was at our immediate disposal. There was no point in referring Paul to Youth Protection at this stage, since his mother wanted help and I wanted to preserve the confidence she was showing in me, hoping to find solutions. She had had her own unfortunate experiences with the system in the past and didn't want to repeat that exercise with her son – at least, not unless there was no other option. The first thing was to find a temporary solution in the family circle if possible, to preserve the child's identity links and avoid any solution that might appear to be punitive. I talked to the mother, thinking out loud.

After a long silence, a ray of light appeared. The mother suggested tentatively that perhaps Paul's paternal grandparents could do something. Bingo! Paul had spent a few days with them over the holidays, and he'd been happy and calm while he was with them. They lived in the country, where they raised sheep and goats, and Paul loved caring for the animals. He truly loved his grandparents, who were quite close to the father. Perhaps his father, who had been notably absent from his son's life, would even visit from time to time.

On hearing this suggestion, Paul was transformed. Initially surprised to find me at his house and somewhat ill at ease, he began to tell us stories, show me his toys and ... open up to his mother. He was thrilled with the idea of going back to his grandparents, and they in turn, delighted to see their grandson again, would come to get him the next day. The mother, proud to have come up with her own solution, was also transformed. For a moment, she appeared to be what she surely was quite naturally and would be again in a short time – a mother who was able to give her love freely to her son.

The last I heard, the mother was at a detox centre, hoping to get her life back – and most of all, her son, whom she adored. Paul was at school in the country in a regular class, where he was doing well and everyone thought he was quite special. His father was back in contact and visiting on a more regular basis.

Paul was back on track. What had really happened here? What role did I play, involved in the whole business for just a few hours? *Establishing a special relationship, exchanging, decoding, and taking action* ... the basic principles apply. Don't confront an angry child or a weeping mother. Don't make hasty judgments based on initial evidence or symptoms. Step back a bit, then approach them and give them confidence, hope, and strength. Find some codes that explain things and team up for joint action. Everything comes at the right time, if we just know how to wait for it and have faith.

I have frequently found myself at an impasse, in a sort of vacuum in the midst of the action, even when all the pieces of the puzzle seem to be in place. Nearly always, after silences, questions, and a certain feeling of powerlessness, it's just like a play: an event, idea, or suggestion comes, usually from the main parties involved, and we grasp it right away. Then the action begins, playing a supporting role, with restorative effects. Paul was angry, or rather he had angry outbursts, with good reason. He was entitled to be angry as a reaction to his mother's suffering and his father's distancing. It was his way of telling us how hurt he was and asking for help, awkwardly, as is usually the case with children. Their requests take many forms and pathways that are not always obvious and sometimes even seem to be the opposite of their real expectations. We need to learn how to listen, decode, and understand their secret language. We need to take a real interest in them and their situation so we can act on their behalf with those who have the solutions.

CHAPTER SIX

The Search for Identity

At this point, let's take a closer look at the matter of identity, which is to the individual what food is to the physical body. Earlier, we considered the question from the theoretical viewpoint; now it is time to look at some concrete illustrations of the search for identity, seen from the father-son standpoint.

Having a father as a reference point gives a growing child a big advantage. For Ahmed, Steven, Mike, Johnny, and Paulo, the absence of such a reference point caused all kinds of symptoms and problems in their daily lives. While all were prone to moodiness and various behaviours ranging from the unpleasant to the obnoxious, the main thing they had in common was distant or absent fathers. These boys, ranging in age from seven to 11, each bearing the traces of abandonment by his father, embarked on a search to find out where they "belonged." Belonging is an important aspect of attachment, another reference point whose absence can lead to a vacuum in relationships that prevents the person from finding fulfilment in life. Children in such a situation seem to float and wander through life, in a constant state of motion, never stopping for a moment. Their unbalanced emotions are expressed in an anarchic way, often through outlandish behaviour and tantrums. Frequent conflicts are manifest as conduct and behaviour disorders, mental problems, even violence. These boys are frequently punished and excluded, unwanted by everyone, intolerant of family and friends – and constantly seeking a foundation on which to rebuild their fragile equilibrium.

AHMED – CAUGHT BETWEEN TWO CULTURES

Ahmed was the least troubled of the five boys we will meet in this chapter. In fact, it was his father who asked a social worker for help. She in turn sent him to me "to answer all the questions he has." The eight-year-old made a good impression, though he was rather reserved. He had no apparent serious problems at school or with his friends, except for occasional tantrums that his family circle found quite incomprehensible. So what we had here was a healthy child who was doing well at school, had lots of friends, and was crazy about sports. At home, his father described him as being passive to the point of laziness. The two of them lived on their own, and his father told me that Ahmed did nothing to help around the house and spent most of the time watching TV.

Ahmed showed few if any signs that would point to a major problem; at first glance, it was tempting to explain the malaise mentioned by his father as part of a normal relationship between a father and his preteen son. However, the father's fears were clear, and we know from experience that a child who experiences major problems relating to his identity can wind up with much more serious problems.

Recent immigrants to Canada, the family had fled a horrific civil war in their country. The father had come here two years before on his own; the mother and son followed later, under difficult conditions. Then tragedy struck: the mother had died about six months before, after a short illness. Father and son found themselves alone, far from their homeland, in a country where they very much wanted to be but an unfamiliar land all the same, with a new culture that was poles apart from their own. The father, a wise and intelligent man, managed to survive, as did his son, who was intelligent and curious. Both made enormous efforts to get over their grief and loss, but at a high price: they were deeply estranged from one another. The father continued to work and took over the domestic tasks; the child continued to do well at school and even made many friends. But it was obvious that there was a deep gulf between them. This was not the first time they'd been separated – the father had come to the new country on a reconnaissance mission to prepare for his family. Then there was the tragic death of the mother and wife. It was all too much, and though their bond was deep, it seemed they had to grow apart just to survive.

Such was the terrible history I observed. The father was clearly afflicted with deep sadness, his body withered, his voice faint – in fact, it was sometimes hard to hear what he was saying, although there was real animation and tenderness in his voice when he spoke of his son. Was this a sign that he was ready to change things and take charge of his son? I wanted to believe it was.

The son, who was quick to catch on, became more voluble with me after a while. He even seized this opportunity to send his father clear messages, stating his resentment and wishes right out loud. I was there as a witness, to be used as a buffer so they could talk. When we broached the problem of the famous tantrums that had set all this in motion, Ahmed said he didn't understand either. They would occur spontaneously, uncontrollably, and unpredictably, just about anywhere, but so far not at school. It was as if he had suddenly lost his self-control, as if some demon was taking over, dictating violent acts and wicked words. He would become agitated and break things before calming down. The tantrums didn't last long, but they were very violent – not like him at all. To look at the boy, it was hard to believe he could be capable of such aggressive behaviour. I told him what I was thinking and he agreed instantly; he didn't understand it himself.

Suddenly everything changed, and he began to give us a plausible explanation in another voice entirely. His father was still in the room, but Ahmed was talking to me. He said that the tantrums probably represented his overwhelming grief, and that his anger served as an escape valve. He wasn't "sick," and he continued to function well apart from these periods of great distress. Once he had explained this, the tantrums seemed more "normal." We now understood what they meant: the tantrums were a cry for help to his poor father, Ahmed's only tie to his mother and his culture.

Ahmed had lost his homeland suddenly, and then his mother. Now he felt that he was also losing his father, who begged me in his own naive way to help and tell him what to do.

After a while, I realized that he was an authoritarian and traditional father who respected his own culture and religion but was unfamiliar with the concept of compromise and reconciliation with his son. For example, he could not expose his body in front of his son in the shower or at the swimming pool, so he could not say yes when Ahmed asked him to go swimming with him, as his friends' fathers did. Such proximity was simply not part of their cultural habits. What really mattered to him was that his son should learn the foundations of his religion. He expected him to read the holy book every day, despite the fact that it was written in a language that neither understood, as translation was not deemed to be pure or acceptable. The son actually complained about this on a subsequent visit.

The two of them were clearly at cross-purposes, and their relationship had become more and more troubled in recent months. None of this would have been imaginable in their homeland, but it was the reality here, and they both knew that. My own comments and explanations (which echoed Ahmed's own words) also seemed to mean something to the father. More than anyone, he could feel the widening gap between himself and his son, who did not hesitate to confide in me, a total stranger, and even used me to "talk" to his father.

Ahmed was being exposed to new ways of doing things, different habits and attitudes that held considerable attraction for him in his new country. He was curious and fascinated by what he saw and heard, the "freedom" his friends enjoyed, the very different father-son relationships they had, and the sheer abundance of this society. He had lost his country and his mother but not his sense of curiosity, which helped him shoulder his loss and work through his grief. However, he could see how much his father was suffering and appreciate the ambiguity of their situation.

Even at this age, while most children can be quite intolerant and demanding, they are generally extremely sensitive when it comes to people they love. Ahmed could not satisfy his curiosity or give himself permission to enjoy new experiences without feeling a great sorrow for his father and a real attachment to his own culture at the same time. He urgently needed to identify with the only person who could provide guidance and steer him clear of further trauma. At the same time, he had no choice but to adapt to this new situation if he was to survive and thrive. Father and son needed to establish a new form of communication as quickly as possible.

Both had come to understand all sorts of things right from the initial interview. At first, my role was to act as a *mirror*, reflecting their emotions and the facts. Then I became the *facilitator*, trying to fix the bond between them, with compassion for their respective experiences, an understanding of the issues, and a sharing of experience and techniques. The father had to play his role as a link to their customs and culture, but he also needed to provide a framework, impose duties, recommend attitudes, and teach values. And as things currently stood, he needed to grow closer to his son while respecting his own values, share important events with him, and come to an understanding of his own mechanisms for development and adaptation. The father needed to serve as a guide for the son and give him permission to make the necessary adaptations, while respecting where he came from, his sense of "belonging."

It was quite a challenge. If there was no identification with the father, no healing rapprochement of sorrows and losses, the child would look elsewhere for the answers and references he needed, the gap between father and son would grow even wider, rejection would loom as a distinct possibility, and the risk of serious conflict would continue to escalate. Without this sense of belonging, the child would be like an unidentified flying object, constantly searching for a landing pad that he might never find.

After several meetings that I thought both father and son found reassuring, I could see that the father's anxiety level was lower and Ahmed was starting to enjoy life again. The tantrums were now a thing of the past, and they'd found activities to do together while keeping the proper distance. For example, the father would now take his son to the swimming pool without going into the water himself and was taking more interest in school activities. Ahmed was now willing to help around the house. After a while, they stopped coming to see me. I still see them on the street from time to time, always in a good mood. They look happy to be together. We say hello and smile.

STEVEN — THE FATHER WHO NEVER CAME BACK

Steven, who was seven, had already experienced various upheavals in the course of his short life. His mother made the appointment to come and see me at the suggestion of people in the family circle, especially her current mate. Like Ahmed, Steven was having tantrums his mother described as "terrible," but his history and trajectory were totally different.

The child had had major problems since early infancy. He was not an easy baby, crying constantly and inconsolably, day and night. There seemed no way to calm him – speaking softly, caressing him, giving him medicine, nothing worked. He slept fitfully and would only calm down for short periods. When he finally fell asleep, he was still agitated. His mother came to believe that he was "born like that" and "something would have to be done," but since his growth and development were completely normal, she stopped worrying about it.

Steven was an unwanted baby, the result of an unplanned pregnancy. By the time he was conceived, the couple had already had many problems – occasional physical violence and constant verbal violence. The pregnancy was not easy, either. The mother-to-be's distress was reflected in physical problems. She vomited frequently, lost some blood, had a poor appetite, and didn't gain enough weight. Neither the problems nor the violence stopped with the birth of the baby, and the irritability factor in the house rose by several notches. The father did keep in contact with the family for the first two years of Steven's life.

Steven was suffering no physical symptoms – at least, none that were visible. His growth curve was normal and he had started to talk and walk at the right time. He was never sick. He slept poorly and not enough, but everyone was used to it and no one gave it much thought. The couple had many other things to worry about. Steven's character did not improve, and tantrums with crying jags became quite frequent at an early age – the slightest frustration would set him off, for no apparent reason. Steven would erupt into violent sobbing, roll around on the ground, sometimes even throw up – and this would go on for long minutes that seemed like hours. They would let him cry since they'd already tried every possible way of exorcising the child's anger, to absolutely no effect. Although his tantrums had changed over the years, the smallest argument with a friend or the most minor frustration would set him off – sometimes there was no reason at all. Now he would spout bad words repeatedly and hit the wall. He had even smashed a hole in a wall recently. He would throw things or destroy them when these gusts of anger occurred. When he finally calmed down, he would feel drained, begin to cry, and fall into a short sleep, from which he would emerge serene and refreshed.

Normally, Steven was an adorable sociable child who made friends easily. When he came to see me, although I sensed that he was a little sad, he was good company, expressing himself well in a soft voice. No problems had been reported at school, and he never had tantrums there. His marks were good and there was no sign of behavioural disorders.

But things had changed at home. After living together for two difficult years, Steven's parents had finally split up, rather brutally. The father was not there for either the mother or the child. Those rare occasions when he did turn up were unpleasant and traumatic, so the mother decided to stop seeing him entirely. The child showed few apparent signs in reaction to this major change, except for headaches that became more frequent, sometimes with vomiting or stomach cramps, which were attributed to worrying.

Father and son had sporadic contact from then on for brief periods. Steven's maternal grandmother was a consistent presence for both the mother and the son. Since she lived next door, she was very much involved in all the family problems and sometimes took the child in when things were really bad. She served as a constant guide for the child throughout that period. For the past three years, though, a new man had lived with the family, and there was no sign of Steven's father.

Steven adored his mother. After a while, he told me frankly that he would dream about her, always the same dream. "She's right there close to me, I can see her, she falls, and then she dies ..." The same thing every night, leaving him sad and shaken. That was all I learned of his inner life, but he also told me he was constantly searching for his father. For the past year he had called his father on the phone many times a day, every day, but there was no answer. It had become an obsession, and he would spend a great deal of his spare time playing this impossible game. The few times he managed to reach him his father would promise to see him, but he never came. Not once had he kept his promise.

Steven's big secret was that he hadn't given up hope. Day and night, he was torn between the desire to find his father and the fear of losing his mother. He was especially upset when his mother openly chose another man and imposed him on the family. Amid all the chaos, he somehow managed the *tour de force* of developing normally, doing well at school, and keeping his friends. I was amazed at the courage and perseverance, strength and energy the child showed despite his worries. Like his mother, I worried about how things would turn out for this little boy who was trying to cope with such persistent distress, which could erupt at any time, not just into small isolated tantrums but into major disorders that could have a dramatic impact on his life today and in the future.

The first time they came to see me at the clinic, the mother's boyfriend asked me to see him privately at the end of our appointment, saying he had some things to tell me. Steven's mother agreed right away. He told me his problem had to do with his role as substitute father to the boy – a role he was unable to play for two main reasons. First of all, the grandmother, who was always around, as were the boy's aunts, was not letting him take charge of the boy and raise him as he saw fit. If the child did something that deserved punishment, the grandmother would take him and shower him with kisses and presents, which, the mother's boyfriend complained, undermined his authority. Based on my experience, the women's behaviour was preventing the child from establishing a relationship with this new father figure and developing an attachment to him. It was all with the best of intentions, of course, but at this stage the excessive protection was preventing the child from advancing and reappropriating his own life without his father. When the grandmother was not there, the aunts would take over and play the same role.

According to her boyfriend, Steven's mother posed another obstacle to his relationship with the child – because she allowed this invasive intervention to continue, and most of all because after living together for three years, she still had not allowed her boyfriend to play the role of substitute father, which was really necessary as it was doubtless the only effective way to help Steven deal with his obvious distress.

A little later, when I raised the issue with the mother, she conceded that what her boyfriend had told me was true.

Their relationship was stable, she loved him, and she wanted to spend her life with him. She was aware how important it was for him and Steven to get closer, and that was what she wanted. But she didn't know how to go about it. So far, she had been unable to make the decisions she needed to make to change the ambiguous family situation that was so difficult for her son. So she had made the involuntary choice of letting things go. She had allowed the grandmother and her sisters to prevent the new father from forming an attachment to the child, and she had even encouraged Steven to continue his attempts to reach his father. "Keep on calling him, he'll answer one day," she would often tell Steven. And so she had unknowingly encouraged Steven to keep on hoping. She could now see the ambiguity that was Steven's lot in life, the dead-end where he found himself, and the daily losses he was suffering. She had had no idea how much he loved her and cared for her, and the danger he was in due to the current situation. Now she saw what she had to do. The boy had to stop trying to fly solo while his base was just a dream and he was always being told to seek the impossible. She realized that this hopeless search was turning her son into a shapeless being buffeted by the winds, doomed to a crash landing.

The support process was now underway. At the next visit, I could see that things were changing. First of all, Steven's mother told me that she had decided to move and stop living in such close proximity with the family members who, wanting only to help, had stood in the way of finding beneficial solutions. Most important, she was determined to clarify the situation with Steven's natural father and stop encouraging the boy to continue his useless and devastating search for his father. I suggested a way of dealing with this that had been suggested by another patient, five-year-old Freddie. I told her to think of Steven's father as a magician who waves a wand and makes himself disappear. One day he might reappear, but right now he wasn't there. This magic formula could be very effective, allowing the boy to keep his real father in his heart for the future without either feeling totally rejected or keeping false hope alive. It would help him to deal with his everyday situation and give him permission to choose a second father, who was not a magician and was visible, not invisible, standing right there in front of him.

The child's identification process could now proceed in a new paradigm, with all the ingredients to make it work this time. All it would take was a little help and understanding, finding accessible ways to start the process, which was so essential to the child's overall health, without resorting to artificial means such as tranquilizers. In this case, a small push helped the mother give herself permission to take action and do what was necessary.

The last I heard, Steven was having fewer tantrums, though they hadn't completely stopped. His mother reported that she saw him smile more often, he didn't look so sad, and he had started to develop an amazing relationship with his new father, which she observed with great joy. And Steven was no longer spending hours on the phone in futile attempts to reach his absent father.

MIKE — A VICTIM OF LOVE

Until two years ago, Mike was living in a pleasant safe village about 50 kilometres from Montreal. His family was relatively stable and well-to-do, and Mike lived in great comfort. He had all sorts of friends. Although he was agitated, he was happy, doing well enough at school, and had no behavioural disorders. His family setting seemed to be sufficient at the time.

Suddenly, everything changed. His father lost his job, the family home and all their possessions were gone, and they were forced to move. Mike lost all his friends – including his very best friend. The parents separated after this string of catastrophes, and Mike found himself alone in the city with his mother and two older sisters at the age of nine. His mother brought him in to see me, strongly encouraged by a counsellor at school, for Mike's problems had now become serious. He was sent home from school nearly every day for various behavioural problems, he was extremely agitated, and his marks were on a disastrous downslide. The school had tried everything, including trips to the principal's office and intervention by a special tutor and a speech therapy teacher, but they had given up. Mike was getting worse and worse. His mother was told he had to see a doctor before he could come back to school.

At home the situation wasn't much better, although the level of tolerance was higher. Mike was very impatient and clearly not happy with himself. Tension was running high in the house. His mother did what she could and tried to maintain a certain amount of stability, but she confessed that it was becoming more and more difficult, to the point where she was also thinking of giving up. The father, previously an active presence, only took Mike once a month, and the boy always seemed flustered when he returned from his father's. It took two or three days for him to regain his balance, precarious as it was. Mike had no physical problems or obvious primary attention deficits. He had certainly been greatly affected by the multiple losses he had sustained. He talked constantly about how great life had been in the village, his best friend, how much fun they had, how well the family had gotten along. But he never talked about his father or his monthly visits. For now, that subject was taboo.

As a first step, we tried to consolidate by focusing on his many strengths and virtues: he was smart, curious, and definitely capable of hard work. We came to an agreement – Mike promised to devote more energy to his schoolwork with the help of the tutor and we promised to convince the school to give him another chance now that he had a more structured support system. He also agreed to get involved in the after-school activities of his choice. The contract was valid for one month – long enough for him to gauge his ability to take charge through simple motivation and for us to gain a greater understanding of this situation. Now that it was about two years since he had lost everything, the grieving period should be finished and a new network should have formed around him. Unknown factors were clearly prolonging his mourning and affecting his health and his capacity to achieve.

Three weeks later, he was suspended from school again and his marks were even lower. He was disruptive, refused to listen, and he was rude and uncouth with others. On this visit he finally began to tell me about his father. The weekend after our initial meeting, he had spent several days at his father's and had gone home feeling completely disorganized, even incoherent for a while. His mother had put in an urgent call to me.

His father lived in the suburbs with a woman who had children of her own. When Mike was there, apparently he could do whatever he wanted: he watched any video he felt like seeing, went to bed whenever he wanted, but he hardly saw his father. In three days, his father spent a grand total of two hours with him, lecturing the boy in a tone of contempt. Mike told me that he knew that "my father doesn't love me. He takes me out, then talks as if I wasn't there. He tells me I'm sick." Apparently Mike's visits to his father were nothing but excuses for denigrating and humiliating the child, reinforcing the boy's feelings of abandonment and guilt. Then Mike would come home, chanting his familiar refrain, "I wish I'd never left my village."

Despite stepped-up intervention from local resources, respite care and support, daily visits from the tutor, and greater understanding and tolerance from the family circle, Mike continued to get worse. His persistent problems were now taking the form of provocation, and he would sometimes even threaten to kill himself. One day he boasted, "I tried to kill myself," with a knife, no less. He had also threatened to throw himself out the window at school recently "to get it all over with," he said. The situation was deteriorating. The boy was not benefiting from his visits to the psychiatrist we had sent him to, who returned him to "our good offices," having found no indicators of psychopathology or depression. The boy was sleeping and eating well, and he seemed to have a sense of direction, the psychiatrist reported. The suicide threats were just "false alarms" and "cries for help." Well, yes, we agreed, but now what should we do?

At the end of her rope and fearing for his life, Mike's mother was on the verge of having him placed with a foster family. Mike had no friends – they fled at the first opportunity. He still spoke of his village with great nostalgia. He managed to hide his fears and sorrows to some extent but seemed unable to pinpoint the origin of his suffering.

For some time he spoke in clichés, until one day he told me about his visits to his father's house. There was no room for him there, he was always an afterthought, he was not allowed to use the playroom or play with the toys that belonged to the new wife's children. In fact, he had to sleep in a cupboard on a sort of cot, with the door closed. But despite the mental torture and the brutal loss of his self-esteem, he still wanted to go back – just to see his father. It was almost a case of the victim falling in love with the executioner (the father) at an age when role models – in this case especially the father – are so essential to the child's developing personality.

We had finally pinpointed the source of Mike's suffering. He loved his father so much that Dad remained his idol although he was clearly sick, disturbed, and destructive. But the price was just too high – the boy's own resources were completely undermined, he was stagnating and condemned to live in a state of perpetual mourning. Now that we knew the problem, we could figure out how to mitigate its effects, discussing it with Mike and negotiating ways to reassure the boy. I was aware that he was very much afraid of placement (one of his friends had recently moved in with a foster family and he was worried about him), so we would do everything we could to avoid that ultimate solution. If he wanted, we would meet with the father and try to get him to change his hurtful attitudes, if possible. The visits could change – perhaps one-on-one visits, without the others, could be organized. And Mike could go to visit his best friend back in the village.

Recently, Mike found a new idol at the school daycare, Pierre, a monitor and a terrific athlete who was good at all sorts of things. The boy began to speak enthusiastically about Pierre, which never would have happened while he remained fixated on his father. He also agreed to go to summer camp, a decision in which he took great pride. The way was now clear for a simple healing process, beyond all our expectations.

The last time I went to a meeting at Mike's school, I found that his behaviour had greatly improved, apart from occasional bouts of ill temper, which usually occurred two or three days before he went to visit his father, which he still wanted to do. But the father had now agreed to see him alone and spend some extra time with him. And I was amazed to see that Mike had stopped pining for his village.

The psychiatrist was right. Medicine had nothing to offer Mike. He wasn't sick, except in his childish heart, which made me think of what Carson McCullers wrote on the subject: "The hearts of small children are delicate organs. A cruel beginning in this world can twist them into curious shapes ... the heart of a hurt child can shrink so that forever afterward it is hard and pitted as the seed of a peach. Or, again, the heart of such a child may fester and swell until it is misery to carry within the body, easily chafed and hurt by the most ordinary things."[1]

In Mike's case, the main thing was to listen to what he was confiding, try to understand his suffering and emotional wounds, decode the messages and cries for help he was throwing out anarchically to all the adults around him. We needed to be sensitive to his obsession with the village where he had lived such a happy life. Once we understood the message and identified what was really troubling him, we needed to mobilize the family circle and the milieu so that he could resume the trajectory of a normal nine-year-old boy in need of a father, friends, and idols.

JOHNNY — AN UNREACHABLE FATHER

Johnny was not quite eight, but his medical record was already quite thick, with several hospitalizations and operations for various conditions. He had had a record of truancy since kindergarten, and his behaviour was described as agitated. He had difficulty adjusting to large groups and performed better in small groups of two or three students – better yet, one on one. His marks were decent, however, so the "hyperactive" label had not yet been applied to him. He had a two-year-old sister whose birth he had had trouble accepting, and he was still jealous of her. He was surrounded by a devoted family, especially the grandmother and mother, who had a great capacity for attachment.

Johnny's father had been absent for at least three years, but just before he left there was a violent incident at a party in the house. Among other things, the father allowed his son to be sexually assaulted by one of his friends. For the past two years, the father had been serving jail time for robbery with violence. Since then, even phone calls had become a rarity, but Johnny still spoke of his father occasionally and looked forward to his return from his "long trip."

At home, Johnny was quite agitated, sometimes regressing to the point of using baby talk. However, he kept himself clean and had a good appetite and no functional disorders. On examination, he was found to be able to concentrate on specific tasks. His self-esteem and motivation appeared to be nil, however. He freely admitted that he hated school, had trouble writing, would rather fool around in class than do his work, and had a tendency to give up when faced with any difficult task. He once told his teacher at the start of a class project, "Just give me a zero right away." He already belonged to a small gang of boys who specialized in harassing the girls – and he was proud of it.

According to his mother, he had not been himself since the sexual assault. Despite his good qualities and deep attachment to his family, he remained a hurt child, always reacting in an exaggerated way. Steps were taken to reinforce or rather recreate his self-esteem and help him to refocus. The school enrolled him in a special group project, but within a month the situation had further deteriorated, and the mother called me in a state of panic. Johnny was now having sleeping problems and had lost his appetite. His health was cause for concern. At school, he accomplished nothing and nothing was working. He was clearly sad and said that he missed his father terribly. He was beginning to behave aggressively with his mother and his little sister and could not tolerate any frustration.

Johnny was clearly in bad shape. He was hurt by all the deceit and aggression that had undermined his personality and self-esteem at such a fragile age. Most of all, he was greatly distressed by the loss of his father. He could not explain his father's unacceptable behaviour and the way he had abandoned him. The love and attachment he was lucky enough to have around him were not enough to console him for the sorrow he felt at having an unreachable father.

Children's thinking isn't always logical. While we might expect Johnny to be acting out of anger, we would be wrong – sorrow was the underlying emotion. The anger he showed was directed at his mother for letting his father leave or failing to keep him. So it goes in the heart of a child. That is why we, grown-ups and professionals, must make the effort to understand fully before we take action. It is so easy for us to get it wrong.

In this situation, the only helpful thing to do was get the father to become more involved, even from prison, or else make it clear to his son that their relationship was over. This was quite a radical solution, but at least it would make things clear. Besides, considering the boy's state of health and development, we had to act quickly – with a surgical strike. In exchange for Johnny's commitment to put some real effort into his schoolwork and the activities designed to help him rebuild his life, I pledged to contact the father to help him get started on his relationship with his son.

We discussed the commitment with the child at great length, gauging all the possible consequences, including the unpleasant ones. Although children think with their hearts in situations that directly involve their private lives, the fact remains that they can, when they have confidence, be guided to think and analyze things in a rational way – especially when their very survival is at stake. This is an extremely important stage in social pediatrics, in addition to obtaining the agreement of the parent, in this case the mother.

I had a long talk with the father, who was repentant and felt guilty and ashamed to face his child, full of regret for having preferred his friends to his son and failing to help Johnny. When I described Johnny's developmental block and his stagnant state of depression that was causing everyone such great concern, he changed his mind and promised me that he would get back in touch with his son. He promised he would help Johnny find his identify, or at least give him permission to look elsewhere for the belongingness he needed so badly. He kept his promise. He called much more often and had already planned regular visits to the prison for Johnny. He kept his promise for the first time, and the process is now underway.

Let me add a few words here about parents who are having major problems. We are often inclined to judge them quite severely, especially when they commit shocking and abusive acts against their own children. It's only human to feel scandalized and shocked, but in a helping relationship, and in the best interests of the child, it is much better to move on quickly to the next phase – forgiving or setting aside the events in question. After all, our role is not to judge but to help find ways to improve the child's condition.

When a child is suffering from the absence of a loved one, despite all the sorrow and mistreatment, medication and complex therapies do have a role to play. But it makes much more sense to re-establish the attachment links and networks of belonging and set the child back on the road to identity. Many children who experience behavioural problems, deep malaise, frequent headaches, asthma, and aggressiveness are in search of an identity they have never had or have lost brutally. Our crucial role involves finding the deprivation that is at the base of all these problems, and many others as well. We must employ all the means at our disposal to "reconnect" the power that fuels the harmonious development of the individual.

PAULO — SOMEONE ELSE'S SON

Eleven-year-old Paulo had been living in Montreal for the past two years. Born to a father whose family came from Madagascar and a West Indian mother, Paulo had yet to acquire his own identity.

His history consisted of a long string of violent episodes and various traumas. The circumstances surrounding his birth were difficult. The mother had several accidents during her pregnancy and was the victim of physical violence on many occasions. She had pre-eclampsia, and the birth was difficult – not to mention that the child was neither wanted nor planned. The family moved frequently, and the first few months were very rough. When the father became even more violent and impossible to live with, the child was left in the care of his maternal grandparents in the West Indies. Several unsuccessful attempts were made to send him back to his mother, who was living in the US by then, but the reunions never lasted very long. Each time the child would fall sick with a high fever, shivering, and poor general health, although a specific medical cause was never found.

Paulo was bounced around this way for the first few years of his life until his mother, who had now split up with the father, decided to take the boy back and look after him. She was trying to rebuild her own life at the same time. Paulo was six when a new man entered the picture. A few months later, when another baby was born, Paulo had a strong reaction. He regressed and became especially aggressive towards the baby but also towards his mother and her new husband. They decided to send him back to his grandparents for the sake of their life as a couple. In a way, Paulo was "sacrificed" for the good of the family. All this time, there had been no word of the father. There was no contact with him, and no one even knew if he was still alive. In any case, Paulo's life at his grandfather's was calm and restorative. He was happy there, and did well at school and in sports.

The first time I saw him, Paulo had come back to try living with his mother again about a year before. She had moved to Montreal and was trying to rebuild her life again, this time with a new man who was of Haitian origin. There had been another new addition to the family, and Paulo had to adjust yet again to an unfamiliar world. He was now in Grade Three, and his marks were terrible. He was described as having behavioural disorders and learning problems. At home, the situation wasn't much better – he was in perpetual conflict with the mother, the new husband, and his two half-siblings.

Not long before, Paulo's natural father had called from overseas and insisted on talking to his son, who was completely stunned by this and became very angry. Talking to the mother, I learned a few things about the child's history, one of which was especially telling. She described what had happened in the family around the time of Paulo's birth. I had asked her where the name Paulo came from, knowing that in some communities and for many families, names have a particular significance and frequently reflect history or important figures. "When he was born," she told me, "I wasn't even capable of naming my child … So he was given his father's name." A simple explanation, but not easy to decode. I then learned that she had always identified Paulo with his father. "It's a sin," she said, starting to cry. She had just revealed her anguish and sense of guilt about the child. Now she understood how aberrant the situation was and that the mental association (you could almost say the two were merged in her mind) was a heavy burden to impose on the child.

So Paulo had started out in life saddled with a name that was not his own, a name that was his by default, bearing an image that was foreign to him. Then, shunted about, separated, transferred, he was never able to form attachments or do the grieving he needed to do – for his parents and all the places and friends he once knew. Despite her best efforts and with all the good will in the world, his mother, who was herself a victim trying to cope with painful grieving, was unable to reassure the child or help him with the process of identification. Only the grandparents had been able to provide a framework for Paulo, who told me, once we had the basic facts on the table, that he really wanted to leave Montreal and go "home" to his grandparents – the only place where no one reported him as having any problems. He told me that there he had really enjoyed life, he had good friends, was doing well at school, and he loved his grandfather "like a father," although he was quite strict. Here in Montreal, the father was someone to fear. Existing problems and the unsavoury companions he had begun to hang around with would only make the situation worse.

When I told his mother what Paulo wanted she felt better but said that it would have to be clearly spelled out. She did not want the child to perceive this as a break or abandonment. Instead, it meant giving him permission to take new parents (his grandparents) who would take care of him, parents who were choosing him. It would also give Paulo the opportunity to take a new name with which he could really identify, to mark the important milestone of achieving this unique status and give him a fresh start in life.

A few days later I met the grandfather, the new official father of Juan, formerly known as Paulo. The boy had chosen his new name, and the grandfather had come quickly to find his real son and bring him home, full of hope and pride. This time, he knew it was for good.

A few months later, I met the mother in the street. I was amazed when she gave me a big hug and expressed her gratitude for my help. She told me that everything was going well, both for her with her new family and for Paulo, who called her regularly and was having great success with his real family. I happened to be with some guests I was taking to visit a resource we had just set up (a respite centre for children from birth to the age of 12). When my guests asked why this woman was so effusive, I was really at a loss. What had I really done to help in this case? I felt that I had only been a passive witness to a situation that was playing out before my eyes. Nonetheless, mine had been quite an active and determinant role. In social pediatrics, as in life, what happens often seems beyond our control, but we still have a strong connection to it. While it may go beyond the bounds of what we know, it is certainly something we know how to deal with.

CHAPTER SEVEN

The Search for Meaningful Connections

As we have seen, one of the most important sources of security in a child's development is what we call the *attachment base* – all the meaningful connections the child has with those around him or her. That base is built up gradually through all the small daily connections with people the child trusts and loves. That trust is complete. The child can rest assured that they will be there for all the special moments, especially the milestones such as learning to walk or talk. They will be there to confide in and to share the child's special joys. In this type of relationship, the child feels secure in a framework that guides him or her through life. This attachment sets the tone for our lives and provides a reference point we can always count on. It is given freely and nonjudgmentally because it is based on love. That is what makes it so important and that is why a child who lacks such an attachment feels that there is something essential missing – like a house without a foundation. In this chapter, we will meet children who do not have an attachment base, and we will see the effects this yawning gap can have in terms of their development. As their stories show, in social pediatrics the focus is on protecting or recreating the attachment base for children who need one – if it is not too late.

DENNIS — A LOPSIDED ATTACHMENT

After several office appointments had been cancelled, I finally made a home visit to 12-year-old Dennis. The school had reported the child to Youth Protection for truancy – a history of missing school for no reason. I was asked to see him at the clinic because there were concerns for his physical well-being – he was very pale and thin. Over the first six months of the schoolyear, he had only shown up for the first two weeks, then a few other times for an hour or two in the morning. For more than a month now, he had completely stopped going to school and was staying home.

Dennis lived with his mother and two younger siblings – who thought it was very strange that their big brother had dropped out of school, as we learned while chatting over lunch in the Pop-Mobile. Dennis told his family that he wasn't going to school because he was being hassled on the way there – it was verbal harassment, he said. After checking with our network of reliable sources (whose names we cannot divulge at the moment), we found that this was not the case, and that no violence, "taxing," or major threats had occurred.

I arrived with a social worker, and we had to call ahead and present identification at the door. The door was double-locked and the windows and blinds were closed. The house was dark although it was a beautiful sunny day. It was lunchtime, but Dennis was still in his room. After half an hour, he emerged from a long corridor to join us at the kitchen table. He was rangy, thin, and pale, with dark circles under his eyes, rather vacant-looking, as though he'd just got out of bed. He seemed somewhat intimidated, and answered my quite ordinary questions with some hesitation. After a while, he became more animated and joined in the conversation with more presence of mind. His large dark eyes, full of questions, made quite an impression. Judging by his attitude and comments, he was surprised that we had come to talk to him.

What we were seeing was a sort of apathetic heaviness that dragged down his expressions and reactions, as if he were carrying an enormous weight on his shoulders, which were already slightly stooped. He seemed anxious and watchful, as if he were waiting for something disturbing to happen.

Our initial questions about his personal life failed to lead to anything that would explain the current problems. The eldest in the family, he was a wanted and loved child who had developed normally and done quite well in the first few years of elementary school. The only medical problem reported was migraine headaches, diagnosed around the age of six. He had had all sorts of tests, including a brain scan, to rule out major illness, but everything was normal.

When we burrowed a little deeper into the history of his emotions and relationships, however, some useful information emerged. When he was very young the boy had suffered from terrible night terrors, and he had insisted on sleeping with this mother until he was six or seven. Once he started school, he had all sorts of problems due to separation anxiety (uncontrollable crying, tantrums, and soiling his pants), which lasted several months. His file further noted that he had always had great difficulty making and keeping friends as a child.

As soon as these subjects were broached in our kitchen conversation, and especially when the problems were placed in sequence, it became clear that the mother had finally figured out the meaning of her son's problems. Now she recalled other events that led to revealing associations. The headaches at the age of six coincided with her separation from Dennis's father, to whom he was greatly attached. His fears went back to the time a few months before when a man had broken into the house and held a knife to her throat. And since his father left, there had been various situations in which Dennis had tried to act as the man of the house, revealing the mother's own secret desire to feel protected by her eldest son.

All this resurfaced suddenly during our visit. We were right there where everything had happened, where all these events still hung in the air. Bringing all the facts out in the open emphasized the child's distress and, most of all, his inability to complete a harmonious trajectory. He was far too worried about responsibilities that were too much for him, especially protecting his mother and even his sick father, whom he'd started to see again from time to time. Dennis felt a boundless, deep attachment to his parents, but that attachment had been built from the very beginning on a high level of insecurity. He felt divided and exhausted, torn between competing loyalties to a sick, demanding father and a fragile, fearful mother who was unable to manage on her own. His solution for survival, after so many cries for help in every shape and form, was to shut himself away and take refuge from the "normal" world.

After all this intense emotion we needed a diversion, so I asked Dennis to come into the living-room for a physical examination. He was tense, pale, and sweating, but in good condition physically. Taking advantage of being alone together, I asked him point blank to tell me the real reason why he refused to go to school and wanted to stay at home. Looking me in the eye for the first time, he confessed in a resigned voice that he was always worrying about his mother's safety. His greatest wish was to protect her and stay at home to be near her. Sometimes a very simple explanation for complicated things needs to be stated in rather simple terms. What really matters is creating the conditions that allow the child to talk simply.

Dennis's trajectory was moving and logical, and his current state of disarray was easily explained. He had certainly experienced an important attachment, but, to repeat, the attachment had been based on insecurity, so it was distressing rather than reassuring right from the start. Perhaps the connections were woven from ambiguities or inconsistencies in the respective roles that were already undermining and blurring interrelationships. Dennis then remained attached to transitional objects, including the bottle, at an advanced age. He had been rocked, cajoled, and loved, but the love was uncertain, poorly anchored, and frequently threatened. Then he clung to his mother, forcing prolonged contact, day and night. When the time came for the obligatory separation at the age where children have a hard time leaving home to go to school but take pride in it all the same, he suffered great distress and stubbornly refused to be separated. At the same age, he experienced a major and upsetting drama – but this time he was forced to endure a brutal separation from his father. For a while, he blamed his father for this. Then came a period of relative calm, with a sort of stability setting in between visits with his father and his daily life with his mother and sisters. There were no major problems at this time.

Apart from the initial problems, he had no trouble in elementary school but remained isolated, seeing few friends outside the home and sometimes having tantrums as a way of keeping his place in the house. His mother said that he had never really been like the others. Did he think he was taking his father's place in the house or playing at being a man before his time? Was he suffering from the mental health problems of his father, whom he saw every weekend?

When it was time for another radical change – going to high school – things fell apart again and all the repressed latent anger resurfaced. Apart from several minor skirmishes with schoolmates that involved name calling and irritations, he soon decided to return to the maternal bosom, to the only person who offered a peaceful if distant refuge – a distance that he himself maintained. The attack on his mother convinced him of the importance of his role as her perpetual protector. What a wonderful reason to return to the nest and reverse roles!

Dennis was a troubled child, driven by a deep distress that had long been fuelled and maintained in an ambiguous relationship and daily life that were now being translated into tragic consequences, with predictable effects. Dennis was on a typical trajectory of emotional suffering born from a virtually infinite need for love that was just too much for him. How much of this was due to his genetic code, his personality, his family, his environment, and his parents' problems? No one knew, but certainly all these factors contributed to the distress that had grown subtly over the years, to the point where no one had ever thought to contain it.

Someone could have tried to decode the roots of the night terrors when Dennis was tiny, provide better support when he was starting school, find the real reasons for his migraines, help him make the transition to high school, counter his tendency to isolation, decode the attack on his mother ... Now we had to do all this at the same time, recentre the attachment in a framework that would make him feel secure, reconstruct his self-esteem, negotiate his distress and fears, and get him back on a more appropriate trajectory, if possible.

The task was much more arduous now, but with patience it would be possible, with intensive attention from people who really wanted to help him advance, rebalance his emotions, divert his energies to sports or cultural activities, and gradually begin to live the life of a normal preteen. For Dennis had now come to another passage that he could certainly not negotiate alone – and probably didn't want to. Chronologically he was nearly a teenager, but in reality he remained a small child.

So what we had here was a child who was no longer a child and who was confronted with a delay that would be difficult to make up, because no one had known enough to take action sooner. As we have seen, various steps can be taken from the time when we realize what type of assistance and support a child needs. But cumulative delays reduce the chances for complete recovery with no aftereffects. It was still too early to know what the future would hold for Dennis, but we knew that he was on the right track now, going to school regularly, and even had a girlfriend. How it would all turn out, only time would tell.

ERIC – ADRIFT ON A RAFT

Eric was nine years old and had been living with a foster family for more than a year. But now nothing was going right.

As his parents were unable to take care of him, he had been in various foster homes since the age of four months. That was the beginning of a painful journey, adrift on a raft with no home base and no destination. For various reasons, he was not able to stay with any of his foster families for very long. Due to external events, the adults were unable to continue to take care of him, or his disconcerting behaviour would cause even those with the best of intentions to flee. It was the same story every time, coming and going, change and rejection. Never in his short life had Eric been able to stop, hang onto someone, or have the slightest hope of getting his feet on the ground once and for all and beginning to put down roots.

One day when he was about four years old, it seemed that it had finally happened. He met a devoted, loving woman, the type of person it's impossible not to become attached to. He still remembered her and mentioned her often – the only ray of hope in his unstable life. Unfortunately, after a few months the poor woman was exhausted and had to give up. After that, the changes became even more frequent, transitory, and frustrating. Eric frequently found himself in a foster care centre, with a vague impression that he was always being punished for something.

The first time I met Eric, he was in yet another reception centre, which appeared to be adequate. He seemed drained and upset by the idea that his history of rejection might be repeated yet again in the near future. Things were rough, yet again: Eric was moody, demanding, resistant to talking or supervision, constantly testing his identity and his sense of belonging or not belonging with every small conflict. He was ardently searching for his foundations, anticipating (perhaps even hoping for) his next expulsion. That was all he knew in life, and he was quite convinced that that was how it would always be.

At the moment he was not going to school, since he found even small classes very stressful. He would become distressed and disorganized to the point of being unable to function and threaten his schoolmates. So he would spend the whole day playing with model cars in his room, until the next cycle of reaction and provocation began. And yet several adults who had become greatly attached to the boy reported spending some wonderful times with him. His huge smile and mocking eyes could melt the hardest heart.

On my first visit I spent some time alone with him in his room, looking at his model cars and making up stories with him. It was pleasant enough, but there was no warmth or affection – it was just a business relationship, an impersonal game. He tolerated me as a transitional playmate without asking who I was, why I was there, or how long I would stay. Yet our conversation was animated, although I had no idea what it meant, as if he were talking to himself. Ironically, when I got up to leave he asked me when I would be coming back.

At the risk of repeating myself, I'd like to talk for a moment about the impressions we get, especially when we venture into children's territory, where they live, and into their affairs. These visits often seem banal, with nothing much happening. As adults, with our usual criteria for communication, we sometimes feel that we are wasting our time. In the long run, we come to understand that something important is happening, but it's happening very simply and it's the main part of the "establishing a relationship" phase. With children, especially children in distress, it's as if we absolutely must get through this phase of stripping everything bare before we can begin something that could help. What comes next is often surprising.

I later learned that Eric had been followed by various doctors, evaluated, diagnosed, and medicated. The neurologist thought at first that it might be complex epilepsy, since Eric would have episodes of bizarre eye movements (fixation and deviation); then he was diagnosed with attention deficit disorder and prescribed a high dose of Ritalin (methylpheni-date). He was also hospitalized and followed in a psychiatric ward, where he was given tranquillizers to treat his sleeping disorder. Eric told me that the follow-up involved weekly half-hour visits, during which someone said "Hello" when he came in, sat him down to play with blocks, and then said "See you" when it was time for him to go. That's how he remem-bered it, at any rate. He told me candidly that no one (even at the hospital) had spoken with him as I was doing – they would just ignore him or observe what he was doing.

Eric had not received any follow-up for at least six months before our initial meeting due to unknown reasons in the foster family, but he was taking medication, with the prescrip-tions renewed by phone. To me, he seemed extremely dis-tant and hurt, impervious to any compassionate approach or attempt to establish a relationship, floating, with no founda-tion and no moorings, as if lost in his own strange world.

My second visit was to the reception centre where he was to be sent two or three days a week to give his foster family a chance to breathe – and try and spare the child yet another change. We met in a large room. Eric, both foster parents, and several regular caregivers were present. We were all meeting here because new and significant indicators had emerged that we hoped would lead to a last-ditch interven-tion.

Initially, Eric was very distant with us, as though he had no interest in the discussion. Then he approached quietly and fidgeted as if to occupy some space. He was here, there, and everywhere, sometimes stopping to join in the conversation.

His foster mother told us that Eric resisted any form of conflict, even "normal" everyday conflict, refusing to negoti-ate or explain when that was necessary. Every time he was forced to explain inappropriate behaviour or negotiate a lit-tle favour, he chose to flee, saying that he wanted to go back to the reception centre, calling himself "dumb" or "bad." Rather than facing facts or complying with family or social guidelines, he chose punishment or expulsion right off the bat. At that point, he would say he deserved to be sent back to the reception centre and leave the home before he could be punished.

Talking around the table, we discovered another troubling aspect – apparently winter was an especially difficult time for Eric, as reflected in great distress and major behavioural problems. Eric hated winter. Whenever his foster family asked, "Why are things going so badly?" he would say, "Because it's winter." All his losses and rejections had happened during the winter – every "hard knock," every expulsion and break-up. It was pure chance, but he had wound up, quite naturally, thinking that winter meant trauma. Could this be a cyclical process in which the child was associating a particular season with his unhappiness, just as certain psychic problems are associated with anniversaries that are traumatic or painful in the life of the patient – or even the patient's ancestors?

Some strange events occurred during this meeting. The most significant, I believe, was his behaviour when we brought up the subject of his natural mother. In fact, he surprised us by suddenly announcing that he wanted to stay over at his natural mother's house that very night. This was really astonishing because we knew that his mother had barely noticed his existence for the past three years, beyond short visits once or twice a year. We remembered that recently the mother had said that she did not intend to take the boy back but would take him on a special outing, such as going to the movies together, once or twice a month. That was when Eric, in an astonishingly symbolic gesture, climbed into a small cabinet and curled up, closing the doors. We felt that this signified his unequivocal desire to return to the bosom of his mother and the importance of getting the security and stability he clearly needed so desperately, once and for all.

From this point on, our interventions would undergo a radical change. We would need to:

1 make a firm commitment as adults to state our clear interest in Eric, provide totally reliable supervision, refuse to accept his self-inflicted punishments, and make him carry
through with life experiences and learning at all costs;

2 requalify the mother who had long ago been shunted
aside, perhaps due to her self-punishing behaviour or di-
minishing herself in the eyes of society and her own child,
and let the mother become a significant person to Eric in
her own way;

3 give Eric permission to form a new attachment to his
mother and others and promote conditions that would facilitate such an attachment.

Now that we had a symbolic display of the child's needs, it
was time to stop getting caught up in his game of being dis-
credited by society, knowing only how to provoke more rejection and discontent. It was also time to approach the
mother. Though she was currently unable to be a full-time
parent, she could doubtless manage to be a mother for short
periods, which could be extended in the future.

Eric had taught us a lesson: when there is no foundation
you can't build on it, and the raft can only drift along. He
had no choice but to send out cries for help, rebel, or take
refuge in rejection and withdraw until someone took the
time to stop and listen to what he had to say. Eric and all children like him experience great difficulties, which must be al-
leviated to avoid the worst-case scenario. When a mother has
no foundations herself, it is easy to eliminate her, since she
seems unable to offer the minimal security and attachment
required for the harmonious development of her child.
Worse still, she may disqualify herself and run away, feeling
shame and guilt. Relationships must be established with
these parents, for despite their deficiencies and ignorance,
love is usually possible and lasting – and that means great
things are possible.

Eric's mother is the only one who can change the course
of his life, simply by showing her love for him. And all his sor-

rows will vanish into thin air... Our role is to spell out the conditions that pave the way for this return to normalcy. In Eric's case, we could see progress as, slowly but surely, the pieces were picked up.

CHRISTINE — A CASE OF COMPROMISED DEVELOPMENT

Christine, age seven, was sent to see me for severe communication problems. There were two questions: whether her physical problems were related to the communication disorder, and whether she should be referred to a resource that specialized in speech disorders.

For the past two years, she had attended a local school, where she had found several people who gave her help and stimulation; despite some improvements, however, her problem remained and her capacity for learning was seriously compromised. She spoke very little, either in French or her native Spanish, and the school reported that she had trouble decoding and understanding more abstract concepts.

Christine had emigrated from a country in Latin America three years before, with her mother. They came to join the father, who had arrived in Canada five years previously to get some education, earn a good living, and make life brighter for the whole family. Both parents accompanied the child to the consultation. They were a young couple in their thirties with two daughters: Christine and her ten-year-old sister, who did not attend the meeting. The father was completing his studies and the mother had found a job that was beneath her competence level. The father appeared tense and confessed that he had nervous reactions and sometimes had trouble controlling himself. The couple described their relationship as difficult, with frequent explosive outbursts and violence by the father. The mother was calmer, a woman of few words. When she tried to speak or indicate her disagreement, the father would immediately intervene and blame her for this or that, criticizing her negative or antagonistic attitudes, and her personal or monetary demands. The situation didn't seem to be conducive to the healthy development of the children.

Both parents were concerned about Christine's development, which they thought was abnormal. They didn't have much to say about their other child, the ten-year-old, who also had some problems, including a fear of her father and a feeling that he was rejecting her. "We've never had a good relationship," he told me. Christine, on the other hand, had a good relationship with both her parents. I observed that she referred to each of them at different times. For them, however, Christine remained a child apart, different, with problems that they hoped we could take care of.

Christine was calm, well developed physically, and easy to talk to. She had large questioning eyes, and her visual communication and body language were highly developed. She followed the conversation very well and played a role in all our interactions, especially when the conversation became highly emotional or when we were discussing conflicts between the parents. She paid particular attention when her father exerted his authority and stated his expectations, when he referred to cultural habits or when her mother showed that she disagreed or blamed someone. Her eyes, knowing eyes that spoke volumes, jumped from person to person as she sat there without saying a word.

I found out that she was just being weaned from the pacifier, and that she slept with her mother and was unable to either fall asleep or stay asleep without her. They told me that she was very independent in her daily habits, liked to help in the kitchen, and worked hard at school. Everyone agreed that she was very intelligent, was not suffering from any rare disease, her hearing was fine, and her potential quite normal. But she had to learn to communicate clearly.

When I began to examine Christine and ask questions, interacting with her and paying attention, I was surprised to see that she had some abilities that were not obvious at first glance. She was able to communicate, even repeat words and

gestures, identify objects and colours. And those eyes revealed her profound sorrow and distress. It was clear that she
understood much more than she let on, and it was likely that
her unhappiness was at the root of her problems. Nothing in
her history or her medical examination seemed to point to a
physical or mental cause. She obviously had difficulty expressing herself and was mute to some extent, but what
could be stopping an intelligent child with a well-integrated
personality from expressing herself clearly in words?

Could there be a physiological explanation, relating to the
brain itself? There were certainly clear indications of environmental, familial, and emotional roots, which can affect
the systems that enable us to express ourselves in words. We
had to find those underlying causes – the children's development and well-being were at stake. What interventions we
should make and how effective they would be depended on
just such an analysis of possible causes, and the steps to be
taken would need to be organized around the whole set of
causes. Language and communication, like other facets of a
child's development, are based on complex mechanisms that
draw upon the person's physical and mental integrity, as well
as *favourable contexts,* and most of all, motivation and need.

In this case, the general integrity of the systems appeared
to be good. The more specific physiological integrity might
be affected, but from the evidence we had, context and motivation were not on the agenda. We managed to elicit some
explanatory information. Christine had suffered a shock
three years before when the family left their country; she had
lost her grandparents, to whom she was extremely attached,
a few friends, and a large family circle. She did not understand all this, and within a few months of arriving in Canada,
she became sad and withdrawn. Of course she was reunited
with her father, but as they had never been close, he was not
a familiar figure to the child.

Once the parents were together again, their marital problems flared up once more (they were already having trouble
in their homeland). Christine, who was very close to her

mother, did manage to form an attachment to her father but couldn't take sides when their conflicts grew ugly, even violent. Under the circumstances, she apparently decided to remain silent. She certainly decided not to grow or grow up, to keep her precious pacifier to comfort her when things were rough, and to sleep with her mother, which may have been a way of protecting her from a father who she thought took liberties.

Christine was experiencing several conflicts at the same time: a conflict relating to her own development and other conflicts relating to her love for her father and mother – conflicts of belonging and loyalty. Changing the situation would require technical support through specialized stimulation procedures and helpers. But most of the energy would need to be deployed on their life as a family: the father's needs in terms of culture clash, pride, and loyalty; the mother's need for self-affirmation and protection; and Christine's own emotional and psychological needs, which she had borne on her slender shoulders for far too long, to the point of no longer communicating.

It would be easy to slap a "communication disorder" label on the child and provide specialized technical support without entering into the complex family dynamic, which would probably explain many of the child's problems. However, this more global and more intense approach involves a great deal of time and energy and, most of all, the concerted efforts of various professionals who agree to pool information and share ways of doing things. It further requires establishing a range of support systems to help the parents and relaunch the processes that ensure a child's full development – motivation, tastes, abilities, confidence, and hope.

All the chances were on Christine's side. She possessed all the tools she needed to make progress and eventually start talking. Her parents clearly had their own problems to cope with, but once her problems were untangled from her parents', Christine, relieved of a responsibility that was never rightfully hers, could devote her full energies to defending her own cause. And that was exactly what happened. Since the family had grasped all the messages and professionals were available to treat all members of the family, Christine became motivated and began to hope that her father and mother would do better and their problems would be settled. She began to participate in all sorts of activities, and before long she was talking again.

BRIAN – LIFE IS TOUGH AND GROWING UP IS HARD

He was only ten months old when I first met him, under rather dramatic circumstances. I was asked to see him in Emergency – he was losing weight, vomiting, and was in a quasi-marasmic state, i.e., failing to thrive. He had only been "officially sick" for the past two or three days, but there was no simple explanation for his great physical deterioration. We were forced to hospitalize the baby to provide immediate hydration and nutrition, fearing for his life. For two months we attempted to establish a diagnosis and find plausible explanations for his state of health. Extraordinary efforts to make him gain weight yielded only disappointing results. No precise medical causes were detected and the best we could do was stabilize his weight. Psychological causes were suspected, and he was brought back to me under that diagnosis after hospitalization for follow-up. Six years later, I was still seeing the child.

The very first time I saw Brian, I had a vague impression of a pale, anxious, "fragile" mother but didn't pay much attention as we were in the Emergency room, though I did spare a thought for how distressed she must be for her extremely sick baby. On a subsequent visit, however, I detected not just anxiety but great fragility in the mother. It was even more flagrant this time: her voice was feeble, her posture stooped (though she was not yet thirty), and she seemed fearful and distant from her child. Apparently she couldn't bear to be near him, except to move him around rather brusquely.

Little Brian had more colour in his cheeks now and at just over twelve months of age was starting to walk, holding onto something. His general motor development was nearly normal, except for small delays in certain fine movements. What was most striking about the baby, though, was his extreme passivity. He never laughed, never made the slight attempt to smile, and didn't say a word, not even "mama." The main problem was still his failure to gain weight, even on a diet carefully calibrated by the dietitian. The other problem, encopresis, or retained stools, had persisted since he left the hospital.

These remained the major manifestations of Brian's problems for four or five years. There were no further hospitalizations or illnesses, apart from the weight problem and the encopresis, for which there were innumerable visits and consultations that didn't really change anything. We kept coming up against the child's total resistance. While we did see some small fleeting successes, there were many setbacks, too.

Brian's growth curve over the years (see Figure 7) was amazing, resembling a gently sloped staircase with very high steps. Growth came to a standstill several times, as if Brian were hibernating for days or even weeks, and his weight refused to budge. In the beginning, everyone would worry and attempt to find complicated explanations. Then suddenly, on the next visit, he would have gained a few grams and we would relax ... until the next time it happened.

With the stool retention problem, what we gained one day with mineral oil treatment, drugs, or enemas would be lost the next as the child had no bowel movements for several days. Then we would find him all bloated, with large stools palpable throughout the intestines, seemingly more passive than ever. He practically never cried, except during examinations that caused discomfort. When he was afraid, he would take refuge with a toy in the corner but never went to his mother for consolation or protection. Quite the opposite – I never saw his mother make the slightest movement to soothe or reassure the child, let alone help him through these or-

Figure 7
Growth Curve

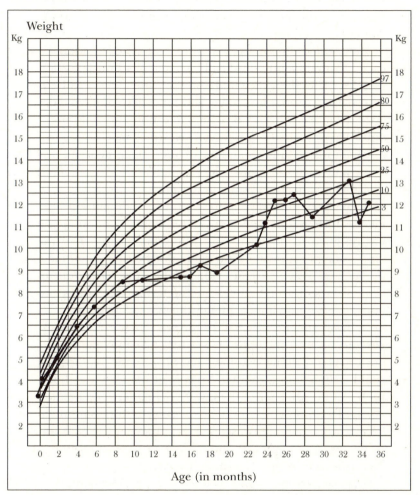

Weight

deals. She let him muddle through on his own. Sometimes she would help me hold him down while I was examining him, but at this time there was not a word or gesture to the child that I could see.

After several follow-up visits, we had reached what we called "a therapeutic dead-end" (that shows how powerless we felt). I feared for the child who now, after a few small successes, had a serious weight lag and some developmental disorders, mainly in terms of communication and fine motor skills. Then suddenly, one crucial fact struck me, leading to a much-improved understanding of the phenomena at play here, and a more appropriate therapeutic orientation. It took a long time, but eventually it came.

What struck me was plain to see: the mother and son were identical. He was an exact copy of his mother, or perhaps he was resigned to mimicking his role model – they had the same strange expressions, the same distress, the same fragility. It was that extreme vulnerability that accumulates through a series of traumas and suffering that is just too much to bear. And it is frequently the mark of great unhappiness, mistreatment, betrayal, or torture. These traumatic experiences set off disruptive waves that make people fragile, like a piece of china that has been broken and reglued but could shatter into a thousand pieces at the slightest shock. Both had the same air of fragility. Now I understood that too much of a rapprochement between them at this point might have had irreparable consequences. Distance was their way of protecting themselves and staying in contact, although their connection was astonishingly weak.

Some steps were taken to attempt a rapprochement, however. The Youth Protection network provided services, as well as health-care professionals and psychologists, to help the mother develop more parenting skills. We did everything possible to promote the mother-child relationship and develop her parenting abilities. For a long time she stayed in a group home with her son, then in supervised housing and with a respite family. For a while Brian was placed with a temporary foster family and mother-child contact was curtailed, but we tried everything to model appropriate contacts. Professionals spared no effort to put this family back together.

Even the court system and the Youth Court became involved, trying to help them despite the sometimes contradictory or conflicting recommendations made by various professionals. Some said firmly that it was time to give up the battle and take the child away from the mother, who was deemed inadequate if not dangerous. Others were still hoping to put their energies into protecting the fragile existing bond between mother and child and making it stronger over time. These decisions and orientations are invariably difficult, and there is no way to say at this point who is right and who is wrong – it all depends on your point of view. To make the most enlightened decision in the best interests of the child, we need to be aware of all aspects of a problem, especially aspects that imply proximity with the people in the case. We must be able to predict what could happen in various cases, as well as the long-term consequences, if possible.

In Brian's case, we did establish special contact with the mother. The child was kept under constant surveillance, and various measures were taken to ensure that he made slow but steady progress. We began to feel hopeful. On the other hand, we had no way of knowing the risks entailed in a complete separation, which was a real possibility and could be more harmful to the child's development than the current situation.

The mother's extreme fragility was of great concern. The subject could not even be broached with her until we had established a relationship over several months. The woman was very young and poor. She had been rejected by her family and had left home around the age of fourteen after suffering various traumas in terms of physical and sexual abuse. Then it was a struggle just to survive. Her general condition was appalling, and she was barely getting by, usually alone in the world. At a certain point what she wanted most in the world began to happen. She wanted to create a real family, and she became pregnant with Brian. But she realized while she was pregnant that she was simply adding another heavy burden to her life. Her pregnancy was difficult: she didn't gain enough weight and couldn't keep any food down. When the baby was born by Caesarean section ("He didn't want to come out," she said), she was unable to hold him. When the nurse brought her the baby, she didn't believe it was hers. Then she grew resigned and made great efforts to be a real mother. But the harder she tried the worse things got, so she distanced herself from the child. That was the pattern until Brian was hospitalized.

After revealing these secrets, the mother opened up even more and told us much more clearly how she felt about her problems. She learned to clarify her needs and even "control" the help everyone was giving her with the best will in the world, which previously she had accepted indiscriminately. She even went so far as to explain and decode what had happened in her life every time Brian stopped gaining weight. Every plateau in the growth curve had an explanation attached to it, which she remembered in detail, and every time coincided with a period of heightened emotion. It may have been some frustration that upset her for some time, or some change in her life that caused a disruption in her habits and a change in behaviour. Then the mother's instability would automatically lead to a crisis for the child, who would lose weight or have another episode of stool retention. With the mother, we revised Brian's growth curve, adding the explanations she gave us (see Figure 8).

Despite the apparent coolness in this woman's relationship with her son and the great distance between them, every little event, every small sorrow or anger, every change was shared in the most intimate way, to the point of harming one as it had harmed the other – especially the child, who was finding life very difficult indeed. It was exactly this symbiotic and destructive relationship we had to work on, now that we had recognized the problem and pinpointed the cause. That is exactly what we did and have continued to do in this case.

Figure 8
Growth Curve Revisited with the Mother

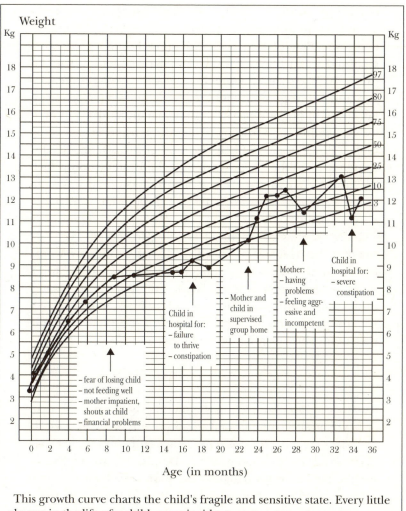

This growth curve charts the child's fragile and sensitive state. Every little change in the life of a child, every incident, every annoyance, every sorrow, is liable to influence his or her development and growth.

Over the years, we have also managed to establish a relationship with Brian. Contact was difficult in the beginning, but he gradually seemed to become resigned, especially when it came to being examined. He agreed to play ball, at first alone, then playing catch with me. It became a sort of established ritual on each visit – our way of getting back in touch. With a great deal of help at daycare, from respite families and a devoted nurse and teachers, he seemed to regain his desire to live and began to smile, laugh loudly, and even let us take him in our arms. When the tension level was too high at home, we would help the mother relax or arrange for respite care so the negative mother-child interaction, which had a tendency to resurface at such times, would stop, and they developed a relationship that gave Brian a stronger sense of security.

Today, seven-year-old Brian is going to school. He's still small for his age, but he's healthy. He has no digestive problems and no major development problems, except for a slight speech impediment. He is still highly emotional, rather immature, and intolerant of change, but he makes friends and is able to express affection. Despite his fragile start in life, he's growing up and living a full life.

AMELIA – DECIDING TO DIE

Amelia's father had been in the waiting-room for more than an hour, after missing several appointments. He had been referred to me but did not have much faith – there had just been too many disappointments. Despite his great concern for the health of his daughter, he didn't really believe that anyone could help. It took me a while to find him, but there he was, pushing his daughter back and forth in her stroller, fast asleep. She soon woke up and screamed the whole time I was talking to her father.

He told me that she had stopped developing at the age of one year. She was now three and a half. Before that, he said, she was a happy, lively, curious child. She was even quite precocious. At the age of one she had a multiword vocabulary, was walking unaided, and was always smiling, he told me tearfully. Then everything came to an abrupt halt, as if the pendulum had swung and time had been suspended. Amelia made no more progress – there were no more smiles, no more happy milestones, just tears and sadness for the father.

Amelia appeared to be an irritable, malnourished, distressed child, her features twisted by fear or pain, impossible to approach and absolutely inconsolable. Her father said her only moments of calm were at home, when he took her in his arms and hummed a few old songs from his homeland far away. But that was a rare occurrence, because he didn't have much time to spend with her and he was the only one taking care of her. What about the mother? "That woman is cold," he said. She had lost interest in the child because Amelia was his favourite, but she was extremely attached to her newborn and gave him all her attention. He explained that since the new baby arrived, Amelia had grown even worse.

When next I saw them on a home visit, it was clear that the child had been abandoned by her offended mother and retrieved in desperation by her remorseful father. She spent most of her time in her bed or sitting in a rocking-chair alone, absorbed in secret thoughts. She seemed to have decided to stop living. Her form of suicide was to stop laughing, playing, talking, or growing up. Her only consolation or relief from violent weeping was to seek solace from her pacifier or a brief respite in her father's arms. After such a break, she would get a second wind and resume her cries of anger and sadness. She barely ate, apart from the occasional bottle, and stayed up all night. The only voice she recognized was her father's. Her mother was foreign to her, and so was her new baby brother. Strangers made her even more irritated. Rarely if ever had I seen a child so deprived, in such anguish, and so resistant to the slightest approach or contact. She seemed to be completely determined to block her development and put an end to this dull life of hers.

A little while before, she had been investigated at the hospital for loss of appetite and delayed growth but released without a precise diagnosis after having several tests. The only explanation for such serious phenomena with such grave consequences would be great emotional suffering, or what we call pervasive developmental disorder.

The emotional suffering of a three-year-old cannot be quantified, but it is not acceptable in a society that seeks to protect and promote the development of children. It is difficult for all of us, powerless in the face of a despairing child, to imagine what suffering such despair can generate.

The family was obviously in deep trouble. Previous attempts to provide support had ended in blunt refusal when the professional tried to ask more intimate questions. Among other things, there seemed to have been violence in the family. A huge gulf had formed and no intervention had been able to bridge the gap. The mother escaped to a shelter several times, but always went home ... for the children. We realized that the mother had felt obliged to make a terrible choice and resigned herself to abandoning Amelia for her own protection. In the face of such sorrow, the child had no way out but to dissociate herself from all this pain and just give up, hoping to leave a world that seemed so hostile. What choice did she have but to stop eating, cry her eyes out, stop growing, fall sick, and let herself die?

A hopeless child in a situation that is just too painful can only use her body and her feelings to cry out for help. We saw this with Brian, and the same was true for Amelia. After a certain point it is too late, and there is little we can offer to console these children.

Amelia was now suffering from many ills. She had a severe attachment problem, abandoned to herself more than two years before. She had a major developmental problem, was not making any progress, and was blocking all attempts at communication. She had stopped growing and did not have the resources to survive much longer. What could anyone do?

CHAPTER EIGHT

An Effective Approach: Further Considerations

As we've seen, the EEDA approach really is quite different. It gets children – children who really need help – back on track and gives us effective tools to use to help them. The approach provides an overview of children in their natural surroundings, an understanding of the set of factors that affect their health and well-being, and sustained action from a network comprising the community and the family.

The steps we take are first and foremost centred *on the child*, his or her personality, experience, capabilities, and aspirations. Then we work actively:

1 *on the child's family*, living conditions, origins, and expectations;
2 *on the child's natural surroundings*: daycare, school, neighbours, recreation centres;
3 *on the child's community*, activities, standards, responsibilities, limitations, and autonomy;
4 *on society* itself: values, views on children, and ethics.

The underlying principle of social pediatrics is showing *respect* for individuals and communities, which not only facilitates what we do but also boosts the effectiveness of the support we provide for the child and the development of the structural bases that are so essential to every child's health and harmonious development.

Social pediatrics interventions are designed to give children access to all the resources they need to build a harmonious life in their own circle on every level – physical, mental, intellectual, emotional, and spiritual. The objective is to help build the foundations that are essential to their development, from a perspective of continuity and based on a dynamic process. These vital foundations relate to physical health, identity, stability, and security – all fundamental rights of children. Sad to say, those rights are far from universally respected today, as we settle into the third millennium. To illustrate the importance of those rights, let's meet some children whose stories really speak for themselves.

THE RIGHT TO PHYSICAL SAFETY

This right includes all the conditions for physical integrity and the harmonious growth of the individual – everything from the quality of the air we breathe and the water we drink to the quantity and quality of the food we eat. It also includes healthy living conditions, hygiene, adequate housing, and preventive tools, such as access to vaccination and basic health care. All of these must be freely available to all the children of the world. This responsibility is shared by the family and the community in a society that considers its children to be of high importance.

Andrew – A Simple Problem

Andrew had been sent to the principal's office before the first bell rang that morning. His kindergarten teacher noticed that Andrew looked very pale and tired and was worried about the child's health. I was asked to see him since I happened to be at the school for a parents' meeting. Andrew was five but so small and frail most people would take him for a three- or four-year-old. He really did look sick that morning. He looked malnourished, and he was pale and sweaty, with deep circles under his eyes. He said he had a

tummy ache, but on examination I could find nothing particular – at least, no infection or acute condition.

Noticing the smell of acetone on his breath, I initially suspected diabetes or a blood sugar problem. I was about to ver-
ify my hypothesis when a teacher who knew the family
suggested a simpler, more straightforward diagnosis: the
chronic lack of food in this extremely poor household. In
fact, not only had the boy not eaten breakfast that morning,
all he'd had for at least three days was two slices of bread with
a smear of peanut butter and some water. I had to pinch myself – was this happening in an underdeveloped country at a
time of great famine? No, this was an elementary school in
Montreal in the late 1990s.

When we took the boy home, we saw a picture of desola-
tion. The mother had no money at all. She was alone with
two other small children in a cold run-down apartment. The
pantry and fridge were empty, and it would be another week
before the welfare cheque arrived. The simplest diagnosis
was right. In this extreme case, not even the most basic needs
that would let a child get through the day, grow, and thrive
were being filled. It was certainly not the poor mother's fault,
as some might believe. A victim herself, she had sufficient
maternal instinct to deprive herself completely so that the
children could have what little food there was.

The child's right to healthy living conditions and a nutritious diet is an inalienable and unconditional basic right in a
healthy community. For Andrew, that right was purely theoretical.

THE RIGHT TO SECURITY

For a child, safe and secure living conditions are a very basic
right. The right to security puts children in the right frame
of mind to grow up in a harmonious way. It also maintains
the integrity of the individual and provides pointers to development. A child who enjoys the right to security is able to
develop and progress through life in the absence of violence

or threats. The child can trust that he or she will receive guidance and clear signals to follow along the way. Security also means having the opportunity to live in a just world that keeps an eye on the child and is always there for a child who needs help. An anxious, insecure child can easily become distressed and act out, with behaviour designed to provoke and make life difficult for those in the child's circle. The result is frequently compromised development.

Sabrina – Still a Little Girl

Sabrina was fifteen, with a mental age of seven or eight in terms of certain aspects of her development. I had known her since the age of seven, when she was brought to my clinic for an eye problem. Knowing her background, we wondered whether she had been the victim of violence, but it turned out to be only an infection. I saw her again when she began to have problems at school – as early as first grade, she seemed to be unable to understand or learn. School became a nightmare for Sabrina. Being unable to learn like the others set her apart from her schoolmates, she often told me tearfully. At first glance you might suspect some form of intellectual delay, but although she certainly had some limitations, the more we came to know her the less we felt that hypothesis was plausible. In fact, we often felt her problem was immaturity and a deep sense of insecurity. She was also good at hiding deeper problems and taking refuge in regression, which would also explain her difficulties. Personally, I never believed she had a real disability.

Sabrina lived with her mother, who usually took in a boarder to help pay the rent. When I made my house calls I could clearly see the level of insecurity in the home. The mother was overprotective and distrustful, trying to cope with her own mental health problems. The apartment was dark and sparsely furnished. The boarder was definitely cause for concern – but a great help in making ends meet, said the mother. Over the years, Sabrina had all sorts of problems. It was difficult, if not impossible, to understand what was behind most of her problems, though her compulsive mother documented them in great detail. Sometimes she would refuse to take a bath (she was afraid of the bathroom), or she wet her bed, or suffered from constipation. Sometimes it was a phobia, such as refusing to go out, or sleeping problems.

An insecure home, dubious influences and role models, and hidden hurts combined to prevent Sabrina from growing up and learning. Everyone who had contact with the child tried to help her, and we met frequently to find new ways to help. We approached her, gradually establishing a relationship. We gave her responsibilities and helped her get into recreational activities and camps. But just as we felt she was on the verge of confiding in us, her mother would present an obstacle, moving the family or getting sick again herself. This would displace the problem and prevent any intervention on our part. It was becoming more and more obvious that the mother's problems were transposed to the daughter and that she had total control over Sabrina. But that was not enough to explain the child's problems and why they persisted despite all the help she was getting.

When Sabrina was thirteen, we managed to give her a few days' respite while her mother was in the hospital. She wrote a very sad letter expressing her distress, sorrow, and deep insecurity. She described how she had been mistreated since a very early age. And it was still happening – first it was an uncle she detested, then friends of her mother's, and then most of the boarders who lived with them. She said that her mother had to tolerate the sexual abuse for fear of losing everything. Sabrina never renounced the letter but made us promise to keep it secret until she was ready to testify in court.

Our initial impression had been correct. But why had she taken so long to tell us? Why wait so long for these abominations to end? There were several significant people in her life she could trust. The reason was clear: she lived in perpetual fear – fear of displeasing her abusers and fear of hurting her poor mother and losing her forever. In this climate of total insecurity, where she had everything to lose, she could only regress, remain a little girl, and refuse to grow up and become a woman.

A few months later, I was called as a witness in the case. Sabrina wanted me to be there, along with another professional with whom she had become very close, to testify to the courageous step she had taken. We were very proud of her, and we had told her so. When it was my turn to take the stand, with Sabrina looking on, I said that I had great confidence in this child, who had been my patient for years. I said that the changes in her life that we all hoped to see (as did Sabrina herself) would certainly contribute to her development, and that I had complete faith in her and always would have. She burst into tears and later thanked me again and again for my testimony. "It was so touching. I'll never forget it," she told me.

For a few months she lived apart from her mother, still feeling guilty as her mother was getting sicker. Every day it was a struggle not to go back to her. She saw herself as a "bad girl" and cried herself to sleep every night. All the same, she was growing up and changing very quickly. She was almost a woman now, and she was proud of that. At last, despite her sorrow and conflicting feelings, she felt more secure. How long would it take to heal all the wounds in her heart? What further torments awaited her before she could free herself from all these disturbing feelings? The road would be long, with many potholes along the way, but her healing process would go on. We had set the change in motion, but she was the one who maintained the momentum, through sheer willpower. She was the one who wanted to change, and she was the one who felt the beneficial effects. The process was unstoppable. Recently, she told me how liberated she felt, but she still couldn't help shedding a few tears for her poor mother, whom she'd just been to visit.

Healing the soul and the whole person is a lengthy and complex process that calls upon all the energies the individual can muster. It is impossible to predict what scars and lingering effects it may leave. Our role is to accompany the person who is going through such a process, be there the whole time, take action when times are tough, and see it through to the end. We need to be there at the right time saying the right things, and stay for as long as it takes – until the healing process is complete.

THE RIGHT TO A STABLE LIFE

What we mean here by stability is having the assurance that things will go on and significant people will continue to be there in a context where values, rules, and frameworks are clear and applied consistently and universally. That stability also provides a basic reference point from day to day, which helps children understand issues and limits and provides the motivation for their development.

Stability is the state of balance in a child's environment that encourages the child to walk and talk for the first time and builds the child's self-confidence. Stability provides the energy to face everyday constraints and failures and reduces the risks and consequences of "cracks" and breakdowns. In this sense, it is both a fundamental need and a right for the child, who can suffer great trauma if stability is not provided.

The story of Melissa provides food for thought on the consequences of lack of stability. It is not a matter of sheltering the child from the cracks – things happen, to adults and to children, and we have no way of stopping them. What is important is how we protect the child in these difficult times to avoid breaking the fundamental balance based on stability. The point is to respect the child, not to "drop" the child all of a sudden, and make sure that someone takes care so that, at the very least, the child does not lose what he or she has already managed to acquire.

Melissa – Mission Impossible

For twelve-year-old Melissa, instability had become a way of life when her mother fell ill a few years before. Her grandfather brought her in for this appointment, which had been requested by the principal of her school and their family doctor. Her family came from the West Indies, but most of them were now living in Montreal. They wanted her to see me partly to discuss Melissa's learning problems but mainly because they had observed recently that she seemed to be profoundly sad. In addition, she had made some shattering revelations to the social worker about her family life.

Around eight years before, when Melissa was only four, a disturbing event had profoundly affected her development. The "official" version of the story was that the mother had had a fit, out of the blue, leaving her in a deep coma from which she had never emerged to this day. Melissa, previously described as a model child, full of energy, always smiling, became another person, emotionally flat. She now had nothing but worries, the kind of worries only adults should have to deal with in times of great stress – or sometimes children who are keeping secrets that are too much for them to bear.

Melissa gave the impression of being a mature young girl. She was pretty, intelligent, and her interactions with adults were quite satisfactory. We did not see clear signs of depression or any other mental health problem. However, we could see that she was going to great lengths to conceal her deep sorrow, which made her feel very fragile when it came to discussing certain emotions. When it was time to talk about the people she loved, her sadness, and her anger, we could feel her heart growing heavy and see the tears springing to her eyes. She had long since learned to contain her feelings and not to trust anyone too quickly, so her sorrow was balanced, at least in the external signs she showed. We also observed that she was surrounded by significant and trustworthy individuals for whom she expressed great affection and to whom she was clearly deeply attached. There was her grandfather, an older sister, and an aunt, her mother's sister. She managed well in her daily life, not complaining of any illness or functional disorder, and was in excellent physical health. The only aspect that left anything to be desired was her marks. Melissa was a hard-working and intelligent girl.

We felt that the father needed to be involved, so we had tried to reach him to invite him to this first meeting, but to no avail. The only way to reach him was through intermediaries or by leaving messages on his voice mail, and he never returned our calls. Melissa and the rest of the family also had to jump through hoops to get in touch with him, without much success. However, we knew that he didn't want strangers poking into his affairs, especially not a social worker sent by the school. Even the doctor (though he was a pediatrician) apparently wouldn't do, since the father wasn't answering my calls either. The grandfather told us how difficult Melissa's father could be. Not only was he hard to reach but he assumed no personal or financial responsibility. However, he did have a certain degree of control over the child's environment through his obstinate refusal to let anyone help her, which he obviously thought was unnecessary.

He was still receiving family allowance cheques but seldom gave money to the grandfather, who was the child's official guardian. The grandfather seemed unwilling to discuss the father at great length, giving the impression that he had something to fear. Otherwise, he was extremely cooperative, obviously very interested in finding help for Melissa. He burst into tears several times during our interview.

Since her accident, the mother had been in a hospice, in such a deep coma that there was no possibility of any form of communication with anyone – especially the child she couldn't even recognize. All the same, Melissa faithfully visited her mother every Sunday for several hours. She had never failed to perform this duty over all the years since the "crisis" that was still shrouded in such mystery. The description of what happened was rather vague. Apparently the mother had given a sudden shout and fallen to the ground unconscious. Melissa found her and stayed with her until the ambulance came. Her father apparently blamed her and held her responsible, which basically spelled the end of their relationship. Although her father was her legal guardian, Melissa had never lived with him since then, and he had even started another family. There was a vague idea that there had been conjugal violence for several years before the mother fell ill. What had really happened? And why lay the blame at the feet of a child in such a cruel way, destabilizing her completely? We would never find out.

And so began the long martyrdom of the defenceless child blamed for such a terrible calamity. The whole base of stability and love that had been so central to her development up to the age of four crumbled with the announcement that her mother was in a coma. Blame, mourning, and rejection were now the legacy of this little girl, who turned her despair into the silent ritual of visiting her mother. She continued to grow up, went to school, and never missed a visit to her mother – but she never smiled. She wasn't herself, and over the years she gradually even stopped hoping for more. Like her grandfather, she continued to believe that one day her mother would wake up and absolve her of her guilt. That was probably what gave her the will to keep on living.

Melissa cried whenever anyone mentioned her mother, although she had learned to hold back her tears. But at least she was willing to talk about it now and envision the possibility that her mother would never wake up. When it came to her father, she had mixed feelings. She saw him sometimes when he surprised her with a brief visit. He had never again spoken of the mother. Sometimes he would take her to his house, but she had started to refuse to go. She didn't like her father's new girlfriend and she detested his friends, who she said "weren't nice." They tried to make her drink beer. "It stinks, and they hassle me," she said. "I don't want to go back." Melissa's little sister also lived with their grandfather. I didn't find this out till later, when Melissa told me she was worried about her sister, who wasn't eating well, and asked me to see her.

Once she asked me to talk to her father, but it turned out to be impossible. The grandfather felt that it would be too risky for Melissa, who could suffer unpleasant consequences. After a while, she said that she considered her grandfather to be her father, that she would refuse to go to her father's from now on, and that she really wanted help and needed privacy. We called a meeting for all the significant people in Melissa's life so we could sit down together and make a list of what she needed and what solutions we could suggest for her. Here is what came out of that meeting:

- To meet Melissa's need for *stability*, we told her that we agreed on her choice of her grandfather, and he spontane-ously confirmed his acceptance: she would become his daughter. We would also do whatever we could to help Me-lissa clarify events and get the true version of her mother's accident, as well as clear authority from the father to con-firm the grandfather's new role in her life.
- To meet Melissa's need for *privacy*, she wanted to have a space of her own for thinking, reading, and writing. Her fa-ther had often discouraged her from filling this need. She had no private space at her grandfather's. We agreed that we would make an effort to provide such a space and give her a "secret box" where she could lock away her secrets forever.
- To meet the needs Melissa had expressed for *support* and *company* so that she could refocus on herself and her devel-opment and compensate for her sad, guilt-ridden child-hood if possible, she would need support in grieving for her mother and clarifying her relationship with her father. Her older sister and her aunt, both of whom were moti-vated to help Melissa get back on track, would accompany her along the way. Resources and activities were found to enhance her self-esteem and put her many talents to use.

Everything was now in place to provide continuity in terms of people and things for this poor child who had been engulfed in reference modes impregnated with failure and breakdown. She needed to reappropriate her vital energies and get back on a normal trajectory – and learn to smile again. Perhaps now her mother could die in peace while Melissa would be able to explore her full potential. What needed to be done for this child had now been done. She had the fundamental right to be put back on track by her family and others in her circle, for her need for stability and continuity had been seriously undermined.

THE IMPORTANCE OF IDENTITY

Identity reaches down to our deepest roots as human beings. It is the backdrop against which our lives unfold. It is what gives every person his or her distinctiveness and special character. It gives us a reason to live. The concept of identity includes continuity and security, providing reference points and connections to the highest human values. That is why children who have lost their identity are sometimes described as seeming to be transparent or cloudlike, as if they were floating. Like a boat drifting aimlessly, at the mercy of wind and tide, they are at risk of running aground or being shipwrecked.

All these children who are forced to survive in a cold and intolerant world, the children no one wanted, rejected or mistreated, separated from their families and emotionally scarred, mutilated or even killed – all these children have an absent or altered identity, and there is no way for them to find the balance they so desperately need all by themselves. Their personalities and their daily reality bear all the hallmarks of lost souls. They are seeking a connection to something, someone, some culture, some values that will help them survive and thrive. Sad or dismayed, aggressive or provocative, their boundless need for love is sometimes reflected in violent attitudes that drive away the very people who could help them or give them the love they so desperately need. If we can only find the right chord to touch, they can learn to form new bonds and put down the roots that will turn their lives around.

Ali – A Case of Mistaken Identity

Four-year-old Ali did not show up for his appointment to see me for a severe eating disorder because something had happened in his family the night before. His father and mother had a fight, the police arrived, his father was thrown in jail for a few hours, then denied contact with the family for several weeks pending sentencing. As Ali's mother told me during a subsequent visit, she was in a state of despair, and this was only a minor dispute. In her homeland, people called the police in this type of situation to arrive at an amicable solution, and she thought it would be the same in Canada. But when the police arrived and saw that her husband's shirt was torn and she had a small scratch on her cheek, they hauled him off to the police station. Seeing all this, Ali had a tantrum. In fact, the dispute, like all their previous arguments, was about Ali and his refusal to eat, which exasperated his father, though his mother took a more conciliatory attitude.

The family had immigrated to Montreal the year before from Africa, with high hopes for a new life in this "promised land." Unfortunately, all they had found was a string of disappointments. Worst of all, their only child was making their lives difficult – for several months he had refused to eat, despite all sorts of interventions. Ali appeared to be in excellent health; his growth curve was above average, with advanced development for his age and a high level of autonomy. In fact, everything about the child contradicted his supposed eating problems. He was the picture of health, so why was he refusing to eat? Could it be because of the migration or his parents' conflict – or did the reasons run deeper?

I started out by looking at Ali's attachment, since it was a great surprise to find a child acting so independently in such a situation. The mother frankly confessed that she was not attached to the child, saying that she was unable to care for him or even take him in her arms. That attitude went a long way towards explaining the child's independent behaviour. The father, who was a student, was too busy to be much involved with the child. Only at meals, in a surge of guilt and parental responsibility, would he try to make the child eat – with no success. Ali would dig in his heels and voice his categorical refusal to eat, loud and clear, hoping to elicit a reaction, any reaction, that would show he belonged to this family. This certainly explained his refusal to eat. The situation was real and shed some light on my hypotheses, but the truth would prove to be more complicated.

In their homeland the family had been quite wealthy. Father and mother both worked, they had servants, and a nanny took care of Ali, so he had little contact with his mother during his infancy. The couple's marriage was not acknowledged by their respective families, who were from different tribes, which meant that there was no contact with the extended family. Four years before, the parents had decided to emigrate to Canada in hopes of improving their life. Before leaving, they made one last attempt at reconciliation with their families. The mother agreed to visit her in-laws in a small village with their baby Ali, who was just one month old.

The night they arrived, the baby died suddenly. This made the mother very angry with the father's family, whom she blamed for the boy's death. Their departure for Canada was postponed. The mother, who also blamed her husband for Ali's death, soon became pregnant with another baby, whom she also named Ali as a replacement for the dead child. Things settled down, but she still could not tolerate her husband and had no warmth to give to the second Ali. His upbringing was delegated to strangers, who took care of the infant until they left for Canada, where they hoped to settle all their problems and find an easier life. In Canada, as in their homeland, the mother didn't want to take care of the child – and didn't really know how. The situation grew worse and worse, and it was then that Ali started to refuse to eat.

Various solutions were tried, including sending Ali to day-care while his parents, who were certainly willing to be helped, tried to solve their own problems. Ali became aggressive and obnoxious. He was expelled from daycare for his violent tantrums. What he was really doing was protesting about not being himself, being a "replacement" child, not having his own identity. This was a case of mistaken identity, and he refused to play that role, one that could only lead to a dead end. Clearly, we needed to identify the child as a full-fledged person, complete with a name that he could now choose for himself. The mother needed to give herself permission to give birth to another child – a child who happened to be four years old. The parents understood, and they complied. A few months later they invited me to the house to introduce me to Kevin (the former Ali the second). The next day, mother and son left for Africa to present the child to the family – a voyage of identity.

While this story may seem far removed from our concerns here in Canada, it provides an excellent illustration of how important identity is to a child. This is a universal story. And it reflects our new reality in Montreal, a cosmopolitan city where people from many cultures rub shoulders – all sharing the same needs and rights.

Annabelle – An Abandoned Child

Annabelle was brought to see me by a social worker. Her life was a disaster. She had severe medical problems: anorexia, vomiting, and frequent fainting episodes during the week before we met. Nine months before, the five-year-old had been abandoned by her desperate mother, who told the social worker, "Take her, I can't manage. I don't want to see her again." She was placed with a temporary foster family, but she was going downhill fast, which was why she was brought to see me.

Annabelle's short life had been a nightmare. Frequently left alone, she had not had any special contact with a significant adult, not even her mother, who had major problems of her own and was unable to take care of a small child. There was no possibility of attachment between the child and her mother, and contact between them, such as it was, took place in an atmosphere of great insecurity. All those years, Annabelle was left to her own devices, causing trouble and a great deal of work for her caregivers, and spending time with transient babysitters who had no commitment to her. She entered the world alone, and so far no one had welcomed her and given her an identity. Her only choice was to let herself die quietly by starving herself, throwing up constantly, and burrowing deeper into a depression that was entirely understandable.

The child was pitiful to see. Pale, small, and destitute, she had huge dark eyes. She was a passive child who paid little attention to what was going on around her. According to her caregiver, she usually refused to let anyone examine her and had a tantrum whenever anyone touched her. This time, though, she let me examine her perhaps from total exhaustion or resignation, or perhaps because she saw a ray of hope when she realized that we were talking about her. I found no clear signs of disease, but she was in a pathetic physical state, with a malnourished body and pale skin, and I could tell from her breath that she had not eaten recently. I was worried. What could we do to care for her, make her want to live, when she had nothing and nobody – and most of all, when she was nobody herself? She barely answered to her name, a name that meant nothing because it was not connected to anyone who loved her.

There was no doubt in our minds: we must find someone to love this child – right away. The only treatment she needed was for someone to give her time and attention, and have the patience to help her carve out her own personality and create an identity that would be hers forever. Medically speaking, we could hospitalize her, care for her body, and ease her depression, but we felt that the risk was just too great. There was no time to waste. Any delay in treating the real cause of the child's illness would be too long. Happily, we soon found a permanent solution.

A single woman had been desperately searching for a child she could adopt and love. She had lots of time to give to the child and so much love to share. It was a miracle. She agreed to make a long-term commitment to the child, starting now. She wanted to give her a name, make her her own, and give her everything she needed.

Within a month, the child was coming back to life without medical treatment. The change was radical. A loving family had worked miracles by taking the trouble to give her the time and love she needed so desperately. Yet again I had witnessed events that were beyond my control, in which I had a chance to take a small but crucial part. This is often the case in social pediatrics, where we are privileged to sit in the front row and sometimes play a small cameo role.

A Plea for Access to Services in the Community

Canadians live in a rich, developed country with a health-care system that is the envy of many other countries around the world because it is so accessible. In reality, however, access to our health-care system can be very different for affluent citizens and those who are not so well to do. While access is indeed universal, the system is strained to its very limits. Some services are no longer insured, and waiting lists are getting longer every day, even for medical examinations or treatments that are absolutely necessary. The poor cannot use the private parallel systems that are springing up every day.

Recently there has been a movement to shift the focus and find creative solutions in the community to compensate for the government's gradual disengagement from physical health care and, above all, from mental and psychosocial health care. This very necessary change is certainly in line with the principles of a global approach – but only if it meets certain criteria, including respect for the natural milieu and the equitable sharing of collective wealth.

We still do not have guidelines for providing adequate support to safeguard the health and well-being of children in their natural milieu. The time for sharing and working in an "egalitarian" partnership between professionals and people in the natural milieu has apparently not yet come. A fair allocation of resources between big-budget institutions and small community projects is not yet on the agenda either, but that is the only way to give *all* children *real* access to care. This is the major issue that concerns us in social pediatrics – and this is what we are trying to demonstrate to society at large.

A true shift to the natural milieu for basic children's heath care, in accordance with children's right to well-being and health, involves a full range of services provided on a priority basis by the child's family circle and those in the child's natural milieu. Such a shift is based on the principles of respect for continuity, belonging, and a broader involvement of the natural milieu to meet children's multifaceted needs. It means sharing responsibilities, sharing power among professionals, respect for families, and availability. It presupposes a change in mentalities, the assurance of training for all types of professionals, and the organization of a support network for the child and family undertaken by the natural milieu itself. In the framework of such an approach, outside help becomes selective and occasional, and it is used as a last resort, since the milieu takes charge of the child and receives support for what it does. Families need no longer hesitate to get medical advice in an inappropriate setting that may be culturally different or threatening. This will also spell the end of treatments that are abandoned part way through because no one understands what needs to be done. Lack of access to essential services due to distance or long waiting lists will also be a thing of the past. Most importantly, it will mean that troubled children who have "fallen through the cracks" or have no one who cares will finally have someone who can be bothered to establish a relationship and truly share with them, understand them, and take steps to help them.

The most important resources are those that are active in the child's own milieu and can work with families and local people to meet the child's needs. Most of all, they can take early action at the right time – *before* problems rear their ugly heads. Resources in the milieu working as a network can undertake a range of effective measures designed to promote good health and preventive habits. This also points the way for the ongoing process of enabling parents, children, and teens to take control of their health and improve their health status by working on the causes and determinants of health. Social pediatrics is committed to supporting this type of action and commitment.

Health care is a resource that requires constant nourishment, cultivation, and maintenance, so that power remains in the hands of the principal parties involved, who control their habits and their environment by making information accessible and providing care that is adapted as needed, equitable, and continuous. When health care is organized into systems that are far removed from where people live and divided into specialties that fail to reflect the multifaceted nature of the human being, it cannot play such a role. Such a system may be useful, but it is incomplete. Only the natural milieu can meet the criteria listed above and fully play all these roles – a committed milieu, properly organized into networks and receiving sustained support.

Since this book was written and first published in French in 1999, a community-based project has been developed in an underserved part of Montreal. This project, which is called AED (Assistance d'enfants en difficulté), or HELP (Helping Helpless Children), is demonstrating how effective a local, respectful, and global approach to child care in the community can be for putting suffering children back on track to a healthier life. More information is available at www.infobuz.com/aed

A new book describing AED/HELP was published in March 2004 by Editions Logiques, Montreal, under the title *Soigner Différemment les Enfants: Méthodes et Approches.*

Notes

PART ONE

1 Nathan, Tobie. *L'Influence qui guérit*. Paris: Éditions Odile Jacobs, 1994, 299.

CHAPTER ONE

1 UNICEF. *The State of the World's Children 2000*. New York: UNICEF, 2000.

2 Pearn, J. "Viewpoint: War-Zone Paediatrics in Rwanda." *Journal of Paediatric Child Health* 32 (1996): 240-95.

3 Emery, J.L. "Parents and Children in Art." *Acta Paediatirica Supplement* 394 (1994): 45.

4 Solnit A.J., et al. "Best Interest of the Child in the Family and the Community: Social, Legal and Medical Implications for Pediatricians." *Pediatric Clinic of North America* 42, no.1 (1995): 181-91.

5 Goldstein, J., Freud, A. and Solnit, A.J. *Before the Best Interests of the Child*. New York: The Free Press, 1979.

6 Lindström, Bengt. "For the Best Interests of the Child: UN Convention on the Rights of the Child." In Bengt Lindström and Nick Spencer, eds, *Social Paediatrics*, 36-44. Oxford, Oxford University Press, 1995.

CHAPTER TWO

1 Fasting, U. "The New Iatrogenesis." In Bengt Lindström and Nick Spencer, eds, *Social Paediatrics*, 260-9. Oxford: Oxford University Press, 1995.

2 Nathan, Tobie. *L'Influence qui guérit.* Paris: Éditions Odile Jacobs, 1994, 299.

3 Eisenberg, L. "Social Policy and Child Health." *Acta Paediatric Supplement* 794 (1994): 7-13.

4 Green, M. "No Child Is an Island: Contextual Pediatrics and the New Health Supervision." *Pediatric Clinic of North America*, 42 (1995): 79-87.

5 Statistics Canada. *Longitudinal Survey of Children and Youth: Social Trends.* Ottawa: Queen's Printer, 1997, 44.

6 Renaud, M. "Expliquer l'inexpliqué." *Interface* 15 (1994): 151-71.

7 Andersen, T.F. "Persistence of Social and Health Problems in the Welfare State: A Danish Cohort Experience from 1948-1979." *Social Science Medicine* 18 (1984): 555-60.

8 Goodyer, I.M. "Family Relationships: Life Events and Childhood Psychopathology." *Journal of Child Psychology and Psychiatry* 31 (1990): 161-92.

9 Goodyer, I.M. "Risk and Resilience Processes in Childhood and Adolescence" (1995). In Lindström and Spencer, eds, *Social Paediatrics*, 433-53.

10 Robichaud, J.B., Guay, L., Colin, C., Pothier, M. *Les liens entre la pauvreté et la santé mentale.* Montreal: Gaétan Morin, 2000, 93-143.

11 Rutter, M. "Psychosocial Resilience and Protective Mechanisms." In Jon Rolf, Ann Masten, Dante Cicchetti, et al., eds. *Risk and Protective Factors in the Development of Psychopathology.* Cambridge: Cambridge University Press, 1990.

12 Goodyer, I. M. "Risk and Resilience Processes in Childhood." In Lindström and Spencer, eds, *Social Paediatrics*, 433-53.

13 Buss, A., and Plomin, R. *"Temperament: Early Developing Personality Traits."* Hillsdale, N.J.: Erlbaum, 1994.

14 Garnezy, N. "*Stress-resistant Children: The Search for Protective Factors.*" Oxford: Pergamon, 1995.

15 Cornia, G.A. "Child Poverty and Deprivation in Industrialized Countries: Recent Trends and Policy Options." Occasional papers 2. Florence, Italy: UNICEF, Innocenti, 1990.

16 St-Peter, R. F., Newacherk, P.W., and Hafon, N. "Access to Care for Poor Children." *Journal of the American Medical Association* 267, no. 2 (1992): 1760-1764

17 Committee on Community Health Services. "Health Needs of Homeless Children and Families." *Paediatrics* 98, no. 4 (1996).

18 Wise, P.U., and Neyers, A. "Poverty and Child Health." *Pediatric Clinic of North America* 35 (1988): 1169-86; Johnston, R.B. "Academic Pediatrics and the Health of Medically Underserved Children in America." *American Journal of Diseases of Children* 147 (1993): 514-15.

19 Paquet, G. "Santé et inégalités sociales." Research documents. Quebec City: Institute quebecois sur la culture, 1989; Robichaud, J.B., Guay, L., Colin, C., Pothier, M. *Les liens entre la pauvreté et la santé mentale.* Montreal: Gaétan Morin, 2000, 93-143.

20 Colin, C., and Desrosiers, H. "Naître égaux et en santé." Quebec City: Ministry of Health and Social Services, 1989, 153.

21 Golding, J., and Butler, N. "*From Birth to Five.*" Oxford: Pergamon, 1986.

22 Spencer, N., and Graham, H. "Children in Poverty." In Lindström and Spencer, eds, *Social Paediatrics,* 361-79.

23 Brooke, O.G., et al. "Effects on Birth Weight of Smoking, Alcohol, Caffeine, Socio-Economic Factors and Psychological Stress." *British Medical Journal* 298 (1989): 795-801. 1989

24 Golding, J., and Butler, N. "The Socio-Economic Factor." In F. Falkner, ed., *Prevention of Perinatal Mortality and Morbidity,* 31-46. Basel: Karger, 1984.

25 Colin, C., Ouellet, F., Boyer, G., and Martin, C. "Extrême pauvreté, maternité et santé." Montreal: Éditions St-Martin, 1992.

26 Cicchetti, D. and Carlson, V. *Child Maltreatment.* Cambridge: Cambridge University Press, 1989.

27 Miller, Alice. *L'enfant sous terreur.* Paris: Aubier, 1999.

28 Tsitoura, S. "Child Abuse and Neglect." In Lindström and Spencer, eds, *Social Paediatrics*, 310-29.

CHAPTER THREE

1 Garbarino, J. *Toward a Sustainable Society.* Chicago: Noble Press, 1992.

2 Nathan, T. *"L'influence qui guérit."* Paris: Éditions Odile Jacob, 1994, 174-86.

3 Garbarino, J. *Toward a Sustainable Society,* 46-55.

4 Schor, E. L. "The Influence of Families on Child Health. Family Behaviors and Child Outcomes." *Pediatric Clinic of North America* 42 (1995): 89-102.

5 Bigner, J. J. *Parent-Child Relations.* New York: McMillan Publishing Co, 1989.

6 Gellerstedt, E., et al. "Beyond Anticipatory Guidance." *Pediatric Clinic of North America,* 42, no. 9 (1995): 65-78.

7 Garnezy, N. *"Stress-resistant Children: The Search for Protective Factors."* Oxford: Pergamon, 1995.

8 Bigner, J.J. *Parent-Child Relations.*

9 Canadian Council on Social Development. *Progress of Canada's Children.* Ottawa: Queen's Printer, 1996.

10 Bretherton, I. "The Origins of Attachment Theory: John Bowlby and Mary Ainsworth." *Developmental Psychology* 23, no. 5 (1992): 759-77.

11 Bowlby, J. *A Secure Base.* New York: Basic Books, 1988.

12 Bowlby, J. *Attachment and Loss.* Vol. 1, *Attachment.* New York: Penguin Books, 1969.

13 Stroufe, L. A., and Fleeson, J. *Attachment and the Construction of Relationships.* Minneapolis: University of Minnesota Press, 1986.

14 Lieberman, A. and Zeanah, C.H. "Disorders of Attachment in Infancy, Childhood, Adolescence." *Psychiatric Clinics of North America* 4, no. 3 (1995).

15 Alma Alta Declaration, Health for All by the Year 2000 Strategy. Geneva: World Health Organization, 1978.

16 Convention on the Rights of the Child. UN General Assembly Resolution 44/25, 20 November 1989.

17 Spencer, N. "Partnership with Parents." In Bengt Lindström and Nick Spencer, eds, *Social Paediatrics*, 540-9. Oxford: Oxford University Press, 1995.

18 Ibid., 8.

19 Doherty, W.J., and Baird, M.A. *Family Therapy and Family Medicine*. Minneapolis: Guilford Press, 1983, 18-19.

20 Chamberland, C. et al. "La prévention des problèmes sociaux: Réalité québécoise." (Excerpt from the Groupe de travail sur les jeunes, 1991, Government of Quebec.) *Service Social* (1993): 42-3.

21 Cook, J., Pechevis, M., and Waterson, T. "Community Diagnosis and Participation." In Lindström and Spencer, eds, *Social Paediatrics*, 550-69.

22 Alma Alta Declaration, World Health Organization.

23 Green, L.W. "The Theory of Participation: A Qualitative Analysis of Its Expression in National and International Health Policies." *Advances in Health Education and Promotion* 1 (1986). 211-36.

24 Rifkins, S. "Lessons from Community Participation in Health Programs." *Health Policy and Planning* 1 (1986): 240-9.

25 Collins, C. "L'expérience du Québec en Promotion de la santé." *La santé de l'homme* 325 (1996): xxiv-xxv.

26 Chamberlin, B., and Wallace, B. "Intersectorial Approaches to Promoting Healthy Families and Children." In Lindström and Spencer, eds, *Social Paediatrics*, 551-69.

27 Tremblay, R.E., Pihl, R.O., Vitaro, F., and Dubkin, P.L. "Predicting Early Onset of Male Antisocial Behavior from Preschool Behavior. A Test of Two Personality Theories." *Archives of General Psychiatry* 51 (1994): 732-3; Màsse, L. C., and Tremblay, R.E. "Behaviour of Boys in Kindergarten and the Onset of Substance Use during Adolescence." *Archive of General Psychiatry* 4, no. 1 (1997: 62-8; Tremblay, R. E., Masse, L. C., et al. "Early Disruptive Behavior, Poor School Achievement, Delinquent Behavior and Delinquent Personality." *Journal of Consulting and Clinical Psychology*, 60 no. 1 (1992):64-72.

CHAPTER FOUR

1 Lindström, B., and Spencer, N. "Preface." In Bergt Lindstrom
   and Nick Spencer, eds, *Social Paediatrics*. Oxford: Oxford University Press, v-viii.

2 Köhler, L. "Health for All Children: A Socio-pediatric Issue."
   Acta Paediatric supplement 394 (1994): 3-6.

3 Pétridou, E. "Social Paediatrics: The Essence and the Vision."
   Soz Praventivmed 37 (1992): 1-2.

4 Haggerty, R. J. "Community Paediatrics: Past and Present."
   Pediatric Annals 23 (1994): 657-63.

5 Kohler, "Health for All Children."

6 Debré, R. *Définition de la pédiatrie sociale*. Paris: Courrier du CIE, 621-6.

7 Haggerty, "Community Paediatrics."

8 Nossar, V. "Community Paediatrics: Caring for Children Better."
   Journal Paediatric Child Health 30 (1994): 96-7.

9 Pless, B. *The Epidemiology of Childhood Disorders*. Oxford: Oxford
   University Press, 1994.

10 Haslam, R.H.A. "How Many Pediatricians Does Canada Need?"
   Canadian Journal of Paediatrics (February 1994): 34-9.

11 Haggerty, R.J. "Child Health 2000: New Pediatrics in the
   Changing Environment of Children in the 21st Century." *Pediatrics supplement* (1985): 804-12.

12 Colemen, W., and Taylor, E.W. "Preface, Family-Focused Pediatrics." *Pediatric Clinic of North America* 42, no. 1 (1995): xiii-xiv.

13 Brown, J., Websnick, M. C., Rushton, F.E., Siegal, C. and R.
   Lamont. "Colorado Pediatricians' Involvement in Community
   Activities." *Western Journal of Medicine* 163, no. 5 (1995): 451-3.

14 Committee on Early Childhood. Adoption and Dependent
   Care, the Pediatrician's Role in Family Support Programs. *Pediatrics* 95, no. 5 (1995).

15 Dobos, A.E., Dworkin, P.H., and Bernstein, B. "Pediatricians'
   Approaches to Developmental Problems. "*Journal of Developmental and Behavioral Pediatrics* 15 (1994): 34-9.

16 Liptak, G.S. "The Role of the Pediatrician in Caring for
   Children with Developmental Disabilities: Overview." *Pediatric
   Annals* 24 (1995): 232-7.

17 McCue Horowitz, S., et al. "Identification and Management of Psychosocial and Developmental Problem in Community-Based Primary Care Pediatric Practices." *Pediatrics* 89, no. 3 (1992): 480-5.

18 Slabry, R.G., and Stringham, P. "Prevention of Peer and Community Violence: The Pediatrician's Role." *Pediatrics* 94, no. 4 (1994): 608-16.

19 Rivara F.P., and Farrington, D.P. "Prevention of Violence: Role of the Pediatrician." *Archives of Pediatric Adolescent Medicine* 149 (1995): 421-9.

20 McCord, T., and Tremblay, R. *Preventing Antisocial Behavior: Interventions from Birth through Adolescence.* New York: Oxford Press, 1992, 117-38.

21 Ibid., 253-82.

22 Ibid., 79.

23 Dubowitz, H., and King, H. "Family Violence: A Child-Centered Family Focused Approach." *Pediatric Clinic of North America* 42, no. 1 (1995): 153-63.

24 Werner, E.E., and Smith, R.S. *Vulnerable but Invincible: A Longitudinal Study of Resilient Children and Youth.* New York: McGraw-Hill, 1982.

25 River Dukarm, C., Holl, J.L, and McAnarney, E.R. "Violence among Children and Adolescents and the Role of the Pediatrician." *Bulletin of the New York Academy of Medicine* 72 , no. 1 (1995): 5-15.

26 Wolfe, D.A. and Korsh, B. "Witnessing Domestic Violence during Childhood and Adolescence." *Pediatrics* 94, no. 4 (1994): 594-9.

CHAPTER FIVE

1 Nathan, Tobie. *L'influence qui guérit.* Paris: Éditions Odile Jacobs, 1994.

CHAPTER SIX

1 McCullers, Carson. Quoted in Carolyn Warner, ed. *The Last Word.* Phoenix: Corporate Education Consulting, 1992, ch. 19.